Best

M000311499

DEFY YOUR DNA

How the New
Gene Patch Personalized Medicines
Will Help You Overcome
Your Greatest Health Challenges

STEPHEN B. SHREWSBURY, MD

10 Finger Press
El Cerrito, CA

www.defyyourdnabook.com
www.facebook.com/defyyourdnabook

Printed in the United States of America.

Published by 10 Finger Press. Distributed to the book trade by Midpoint Trade Books. Edited by The Authors Team (www.AuthorsTeam.com)
Interior Design/Layout: Ghislain Viau

ISBN 9781933174860

Library of Congress Control Number: 2013903576

Publisher's Cataloging-in-Publication
(Provided by Quality Books Inc.)

Shrewsbury, Stephen B.
      Defy your DNA : how the new gene patch personalized
   medicines will help you overcome your greatest health
   challenges / Stephen B. Shrewsbury.
         p. cm.
      Includes bibliographical references and index.

      1. Antisense nucleic acids--Therapeutic use--Popular
   works. 2. Oligonucleotides--Therapeutic use--Popular
   works. 3. Recombinant molecules--Therapeutic use--
   Popular works. 4. Pharmaceutical biotechnology--Popular
   works.   I. Title.

   RM666.A564S57 2013   615.3'1
                           QBI13-200003

   09 08 07 06 05 04   5 4 3 2 1

Table of Contents

This book is dedicated to the many healthy volunteers, patients and their families who have participated in any drug study. Without you there would be no new drugs. Without you there would be no advances in pharmaceuticals. You are the ones who are selflessly bringing hope to the millions of patients around the world waiting for tomorrow's advances in therapeutics.

Acknowledgements

I am indebted to:

Professor Dwight Weller who as Senior Vice President has headed the chemistry department at AVI BioPharma (as it was) since leaving Oregon State University. He has taught me all I know about the chemistry of oligomers and the fact that that is not much is no discredit to him. His review of this manuscript however has been as usual meticulous and constructive.

Professor Ryszard Kole, who worked alongside the Nobel Laureate Professor Sid Altman through the discovery of "alternative splicing" at Yale University. Ryszard was Senior Vice President of Research and Distinguished Scientist during my time at AVI BioPharma and kindly reviewed and provided input to this manuscript as well as teaching me more about exon skipping than I ever expected to grasp.

Dr. Patrick Iversen, was Senior Vice President of Research and Innovation when I was at AVI BioPharma, and my squash partner in Corvallis! Pat has been the tireless, driving force behind the anti-microbial research for the AVI stable of oligomers and found time to review and comment on the relevant sections of this book.

Mahesh Grossman and his colleagues at The Authors Team have helped me make the book more readable, and reduce sentence length, complexity and use of too much jargon! His support as the chapters have ebbed and flowed and each has been scrubbed and buffed over the last sixteen months has been welcome.

Merry Shiyu Wang has provided excellent illustrations and has been approachable, expeditious and efficient turning out diagrams to my design, while making them scientifically accurate and pleasing to the eye. Thank you!

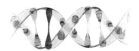

Preface

Some years ago, I was a family doctor in Evesham, a quaint, medieval market town on the banks of the River Avon in Worcestershire, in the United Kingdom. I was getting to the end of my morning surgery when the phone rang. A worried patient was hoping I could see her son.

I knew the patient, Mrs. Singh and her son Deepak, as I did most of my patients. But like most parents, she didn't come very often so I did not know her well. Her son was just over three, and I had looked after Mrs. Singh and her husband since before she gave birth to her daughter Jasminder five years earlier. Deepak had been a happy, healthy baby who had passed his 18-month assessment with me despite being a little slow in walking.

Mrs. Singh came in pushing a grinning and content three-year-old in a stroller. As Deepak stared at me, I wondered if maybe he was just enjoying a little extra attention. Mrs. Singh described how her son had become reluctant to walk in the afternoons and evenings. She was worried that he had hurt his leg or, perhaps, had an infection.

I turned to Deepak, squatting down in front of his stroller so that my eyes were on his level. "What have you got there?" I asked, pointing to a tatty toy he was holding, which I suspected had once resembled a tiger. Deepak beamed but said nothing.

Hoping to entice him to walk, I walked over to a large treasure chest of my own children's discarded toys that were stowed beneath a couch. I pulled out a squeaking elephant toy. That got his attention.

"Look, Deepak," I offered, poking the head of the elephant round the lid of the box and then quickly withdrawing it and squeezing it forcefully. Deepak immediately dropped his tiger and raised himself out of his stroller. He waddled across my examination room toward me - only a few steps, but he seemed indeed rather reluctant. My heart sank. This was not the nimble confident stride of a normal healthy three-year-old.

I gave him the elephant and he sat down with a thump.

I went back to my desk and quickly scanned Deepak's medical records. There was nothing to suggest he was not entirely normal. I quizzed Mrs. Singh about the health of her immediate family, but again there was nothing notable. I continued eyeing Deepak who was playing contentedly. Then he rolled over and struggled to his feet.

With that, I was alarmed.

At medical school, students are taught about rare diseases, but most doctors, especially those with a list of less than 3,000 patients never see a single case of most of them. So the memory fades. But could Deepak have Duchenne muscular dystrophy? It is very rare. It only occurs in boys, often with no family history, and is often undetectable at birth. It could present pretty much the way Deepak appeared now with difficulty walking at around age three with what looked like enlarged calf muscles on his legs.

I got down on my hands and knees and looked carefully at the now standing Deepak, who had become interested in a colorful paperweight on my desk. Certainly he had large calf muscles for a three-year-old. Quite chunky little legs, but were they abnormally so?

This would be a complex diagnosis to make, and a terrible blow to the Singhs. The disease gradually robs boys of muscle power. They lose the ability to walk, and later to even stand with braces, becoming dependent on a wheelchair for mobility. Then they get breathing trouble and require portable ventilators. But despite all the support, they become totally unable to move and often die in their early twenties when their heart muscle also fails, if they survive that long.

Little progress has been made on this terrible disease since it was first described by the French neurologist, Guillaume Duchenne, in 1891. Despite intense study by scientists and doctors over the last century, there is no cure. In 1986, scientists discovered any one of many mutations in a single gene can cause the muscle cells of these boys to fail to make a vital protein. As a result, their muscles waste away. High doses of steroids temporarily delay the inevitable, but no effective treatment existed then or now, and steroids bring problems of their own.

It is a terrible, unforgiving disease, and the knowledge that the best I could do, if I was correct, was to watch Deepak slip away, is one of the most unpleasant professional situations a doctor can encounter.

Therapeutic impotence is something we were taught to cope with at medical school. However, lectures can't prepare a doctor for the horror of telling a mother the devastating future she and her family may face. How could I explain that we could put men on the moon, but I could not stop Deepak from slowly dying over the next twenty years as every muscle in his body stopped working?

Many years later, that horrible feeling remains fresh.

At the time, I thought of my own son who had been born with a rare disease, multicystic dysplastic kidney. He was expected to die soon after his birth, and my world had changed with his arrival.

He survived and thrives to this day, which is not how it would be for Deepak if he had Duchenne muscular dystrophy.

I continued to chat with Mrs. Singh while I desperately considered the other possible diseases, illnesses, and injuries that could have befallen Deepak. None of them seemed likely. Attempting nonchalance, I convinced Mrs. Singh of the need for a blood test and drew the sample from a struggling and howling Deepak.

Several weeks later, the worst case scenario was confirmed. Deepak had Duchenne muscular dystrophy (DMD). The diagnosis was understandably difficult for the Singhs to absorb. No parent wants to limit the dreams they have for their children, much less accept that they would likely outlive their offspring.

Later that same evening, after reading stories to my own children, and marveling at my own son who had miraculously survived the fate that his doctors had predicted for him, I wondered if we would ever develop a treatment, let alone a cure for DMD. By we, I meant all the scientists, doctors, laboratory workers, and everyone else involved in healthcare.

Deepak may be dead now, or struggling in a wheelchair and on a ventilator. What more could I have done for him back then? Nothing. Absolutely nothing. I couldn't even offer hope. That was, perhaps, the hardest lesson and most unpleasant duty I ever had as a doctor.

However, now, in 2012, I am confident that physicians will soon be able to offer more than hope to families like the Singh's. Maybe not this year and maybe not next, but soon. The hope comes from a new class of medicines that can patch the defective message that comes from a faulty gene that cause diseases like Duchenne's. Some of these patches work by stopping the production of a disease causing protein, either within the sick patient, or by an invading bacteria or virus. Others of these new medicines work by triggering a naturally occurring alternative process in the human cell to produce a new version of a vital missing protein. This book focuses mostly on this latter category, which offers great hope. In the future, these new gene patch medicines will allow you to defy your DNA.

My eldest son qualified as a doctor himself in 2011. Because of these new medicines, he will be able to offer hope to ALL of his patients, no matter what their diagnosis. In the not too distant future, when a child is born, they'll be required to have two documents: a birth certificate and a map of their DNA. The map will show which roads to take to get to their destination and which to avoid. Avoiding a bad ending may involve behavioral modification, or traditional medicines or the help of one of these new gene-patch oligomers as they gain acceptance. They are like molecular Band Aids that will hide damaged pieces of the genetic message.

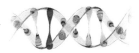

Chapter One

Medicine on the Brink

When, nearly a decade ago, scientists painstakingly documented the entire genetic instruction book for a human being, the human genome, it was a seedling for a new era in medicine. This new era is one where doctors will treat and prevent diseases based on the subtle differences in our DNA.

That feat and subsequent efforts at refinement have unleashed a torrent of information that is just beginning to trickle into physicians' offices as they diagnose and treat more diseases at earlier and earlier stages.

As that trickle becomes a stream, I grow increasingly convinced that the physicians of today, those who graduated at the same time as my son in 2011, will have new tools to treat diseases never before treatable. They will predict and prevent many others. The whole emphasis of medical care will change from treating illness to creating and preserving wellness.

Medicine, western medicine in particular, suffers from an imperfect, but understandable focus. Physicians usually don't intervene until a problem exists. Ever since the first human suffered an ache or pain, our species has sought to alleviate suffering whether through the ministrations of a witch doctor, or a simple brew of the aspirin-like willow bark tea, or in recent times, the newest modern blockbuster drug. For the past five thousand years, medicine has focused on diagnosing and treating already sick and symptomatic people.

Physicians aren't entirely to blame. Patients generally only show up when symptoms appear. Too often that means treating a disease at a very late stage when much damage has already been done. Surgeons have become quite adept at replacing clogged arteries that feed oxygen to the heart, but physicians have been less successful at identifying people at risk for that coronary artery-clogging disease in the first place.

It's not that doctors wouldn't prefer to help their patients stay healthy and well. Intervening in a disease process at its earliest stages is always preferred. Treating a disease before today's laboratory tests or images would show the telltale damage, or being able to prevent it altogether, offers an unprecedented opportunity to deliver optimum health and life expectancy. Doctors just haven't had tests capable of detecting potential problems or the tools needed to avert them.

That is all changing.

Medicine is moving rapidly from a "diagnose and treat" model to a "predict and prevent" model and that will have huge implications for both patients and society.

Imagine going to the doctor who looks at your individual genetic makeup and uses that information to advise you on the most appropriate lifestyle adjustment to prevent a condition years or even decades before it starts causing symptoms. Better still, your doctor may prescribe a precisely targeted medicine for you that will work at the level of a faulty genetic message. So you should never have to worry about falling prey to the condition at all.

This fundamental change in medicine is already taking place.

Driving that change is the torrent of genetic information emerging from efforts to sequence the entire human genome.

In 2003, Nobel Prize winner James Watson was the first to undergo full sequencing of his genome. This effort cost about three billion dollars and took thirteen years.

Now, science and medicine are beginning to harness the information contained within the genome to aid drug development.

At the time of writing this book, there are roughly thirty thousand drugs used in the world. They target about two percent of the proteins found in human cells. This has led to the concept of the "druggable genome". This is the subset of the human genome that contains codes for proteins that small molecule drugs can interact with and affect.

Small molecule drugs are those with a low molecular weight, less than one thousand Daltons, compared to biological molecules that have a much greater weight, and oligomers whose weight is typically between six and seven thousand Daltons. A Dalton, named after the English chemist and physicist, John Dalton (1766 – 1844), is a measurement first coined in 1803 and is set as one-twelfth of the weight of an unbound carbon atom. It is equivalent to 1.66×10^{-27} kg. To make that more meaningful, a small grain of sand weighs about 0.67 mg, or 6.7×10^{-4} kg, meaning that it would take roughly 2×10^{22} atoms of carbon, each weighing 1 Dalton, to weigh as much as a single grain of sand.

Small molecules are chemically synthesized and are manufactured to high levels of purity. In addition, they rarely cause an immune response in humans and generally have the same positive and negative effects in animals. That allows them to be tested in animals first before testing in humans. Biological products, especially the newer monoclonal antibodies, are capable of triggering a marked immune response but often only with a specific species.

Scientists, led by Andrew Hopkins and Colin Groom of the drug company Pfizer, looked into the druggable genome in 2002 and found that a mere 399 proteins had successfully been targeted. Later Hopkins lowered this figure to 207.

About half of the targets fell into one of five protein families: G-protein coupled receptors (GPCRs), kinases, proteases, nuclear hormone receptors, and phosphodiesterases.

But not all of the protein targets may actually modify disease. Some examples within each class may be too difficult to target. With fewer and fewer new small molecule drugs reaching approval, there is great anxiety within the medical and pharmaceutical communities that we may be getting close to having identified all the potential targets that small molecules can reach, and that we are reaching the limit of drug discovery, at least for small molecule drugs.

Since Watson's genome was sequenced, scientists have discovered multiple genes that can predict the risk of one day developing a multitude of diseases. They have discovered genes that can predict how you will burn fat and whether you will develop diabetes. At present, we know of six different genes that affect your chances of developing dementia as a result of Alzheimer's disease. Those genes, however, only play a role in about sixty percent of all Alzheimer's cases. Dr. William Thies, the Chief Medical and Scientific Officer for the Alzheimer's Association, speculates that up to one hundred genes could ultimately play a role.

One approach to Alzheimer's disease is already being explored in a rather unique situation. In the area around Medellin in Colombia, approximately five thousand people are participating in an experiment. They are all descended from 28 original families who carried a single mutation, E280A of the presenilin 1 gene, a gene that causes Alzheimer's disease. These people are at risk of developing the disease not as senior citizens, but in their forties and fifties. In this area of

Antioquia, subjects with the mutation are being identified and tested with potentially preventative drugs in their thirties, in the hope that early onset, familial Alzheimer's disease can be prevented.

Here are some other DNA-related health discoveries that are important: Several genes residing on chromosome five turn out to be related to developing asthma, another common disease. A genetic component has yet to be identified for many cases of schizophrenia, as well as obesity and diabetes. Genes are likely to play a part in whether you develop heart disease and chronic obstructive pulmonary disease (COPD), although a much greater risk is run if you smoke. But if you do smoke, maybe it is because you have inherited the desire, or have the gene that predisposes you to become addicted to nicotine.

The list goes on.

Some diseases are described as "complex" because they result from the interplay of a number of different genes and biological systems, such as your environment.

Cancer is the poster child for complex diseases among those where scientists have discovered that genes confer risk. Because cancer can affect any organ or tissue in the body, it is actually a set of diseases rather than a single ailment. There are faulty genes, named BRCA1 and BRCA2 that increase the risk of developing breast and ovarian cancer in women and breast cancer in men. Similarly, defects in the genes APC and MLH1 raise the risk for developing different types of colon cancer. The ever-growing list of cancer-causing genes is broadly divided into those that cause or promote cancer and those that usually suppress cancer (tumor-suppressor genes). One that was discovered at the Memorial Sloan-Kettering Cancer Center in New York City in 2005, originally called the Pokemon gene and now renamed as Zbtb7, plays a key role in promoting cancer proliferation in surrounding tissues when triggered by another cancer causing gene.

While sequencing Watson's genome proved time consuming and expensive, genome sequencing today can be completed in days and the cost is plummeting towards the one thousand dollar mark. Genetic Testing Laboratory Inc., 23andMe and deCODE genetics are companies that offer a limited service for considerably less than a thousand dollars, directly to consumers or via a healthcare professional.

Many people are already getting their genomes (i.e. all of their ~25,000 genes) sequenced. All it requires are a few cells from inside your cheek that can be provided in a spit sample. Several biotech companies responsible for sequencing the genome have actually held "spit parties" to advertise how easy it is now to provide a suitable sample to permit a full genome sequence. In fact, a party hosted by 23andMe even made the "Fashion & Style" section of The New York Times. A photo of a young couple spitting into collection tubes was captioned, "When in doubt, spit it out."

Patients who enjoy being in the vanguard are taking these analyses into their physician's office to serve as a basis for decisions about their health.

It's at the physician's office where the excitement about tomorrow's personalized medicine can come up against today's cold hard reality. The field of genomics has moved so quickly that many physicians haven't learned how to interpret the results of genome sequencing, which are often quite complex.

Personalized medicine is a developing field and there is a learning curve associated with implementing it. Physicians will be grappling with that learning curve for the next five years, but by the end of this decade, reading the results of genome sequencing will be commonplace for them.

So far the revolution has focused most on detecting risk for disease and many books are being written on the subject. But that is a far cry from being able to effectively treat it.

A doctor who learns that you are harboring genes that increase your risk for diabetes will still advise you to lose weight, especially if other obesity-related genetic variations are part of the mix. However, with a genetic map your doctor may have some extra tools in his arsenal. He may be able to use the genetic information to advise you about the type, frequency and duration of exercise and even the best foods to consume, either before or after exercise, to improve your chances of losing weight. In addition your physician will start more frequent screening for elevated blood sugar levels.

Your physician would be able to advise another patient with a genetically greater risk of developing colon cancer to start routine colonoscopy screening at a younger age and to have those screenings more frequently.

Admittedly, these are today's routine recommendations that you hear from your doctor based on your family history.

But a personalized medicine approach can more precisely define and even quantify the risks that you have inherited from your parents. That may serve as potent motivation for you to make lifestyle changes.

Certain savvy physicians are already employing personal genomic information when prescribing particular drugs.

This will be especially true when it comes to the possible side effects of a drug. Look at any advertisement for a commonly used pharmaceutical. First, you see information about the uses of the drug, then comes a long list of potential side effects and problems you could encounter. Such "adverse events" are common to all pharmaceuticals, and the FDA requires the public to be warned about them. The fact is, we are all subtly different on a genetic level. For some of us, the drug is ineffective. For others, the drug is perhaps harmful. For most, we hope to get a Goldilocks effect where the drug works just right. With modern genomic sequencing, we will be able to tell you whether the drug will provide the required beneficial effects and if those effects will come with harmful side effects.

Take the blood-thinning drug Coumadin, one of the trade names for a drug called warfarin. It's one of the most widely prescribed pharmaceuticals in the United States. Doctors use it to prevent potentially fatal blood clots from forming or growing in blood vessels. People with irregular heartbeats, those who have suffered a heart attack, or those who have had blood clots in their lungs or legs often take the drug.

Warfarin is a lifesaver for many. However, it can have devastating side effects. It is one of the top three drugs associated with emergency room visits in the United States. It has been estimated to cause 85,000 serious bleeds and 17,000 hemorrhagic strokes as well as other adverse drug reactions every year in the U.S. at a cost of one billion dollars.

What makes it so helpful and yet so dangerous at the same time? The genetic makeup of the patients who are taking it is the answer.

You may have genes that break the drug down very slowly, letting too much warfarin into your bloodstream, so that your blood does not clot at all. In that case, you could suffer from life-threatening bleeding. For you, the drug works "too well."

On the other hand, you could break down the drug so quickly that very little ends up in your bloodstream, so it won't actually prevent clots from forming. Warfarin won't work for you.

Doctors can test for the genes responsible for these different responses before prescribing warfarin. They can also now test for genes that affect how well certain antidepressants, painkillers, cancer drugs, blood pressure medications, and other pharmaceuticals work. The tests aren't yet routine and are often only conducted once you have had some problem with a particular drug. But, with the costs of sequencing declining and expected to decline further in the next decade or two, we will all carry electronic versions of our genomes like a credit card in our wallets, on a key fob, or in some as yet unimagined form so that medicines prescribed to us can be more assuredly predicted to be both safe and effective.

When you weed the garden, you must get hold of the weed's root to be successful. That holds for efforts to treat illness too. I doubt there will ever be weed-free gardens. Nor will we ever eliminate all diseases even once the power to predict and prevent has been fully developed. But any disease is best tackled as close to the source as possible, which, in most cases, is our genes.

This isn't a new idea. Scientists have been trying for decades to develop gene therapy approaches that would simply replace faulty DNA and avoid disease entirely. However, getting new genes reliably into cells has so far eluded our best efforts. Perhaps the next best option is to camouflage the faulty messages coming from mutant genes from the rest of the cell. If the faulty part of the message isn't "seen" by the cell's protein making machinery, the defective genetic information can't cause problems. If the protein making machinery, the ribosome, sees something else, something better, the gene's message will have been camouflaged, and the cell will build a protein according to what it sees.

When that happens, the previously inevitable disease will be avoided.

This remarkably simple concept is inspiring an entirely new field of work in the pharmaceutical industry.

Tricking the body into ignoring faulty genetic instructions doesn't require complex efforts to insert new genetic material or delete faulty DNA. It can be accomplished by using drugs made from building blocks remarkably similar to naturally occurring genetic material, the DNA itself. These drugs can camouflage or patch parts of the message that come from our genes. This will stop the cell producing a disease-causing protein, or allow a healthy version of the message to be delivered, rather than a faulty one. If a healthy message is delivered to the cellular machinery carrying vital blueprints, a missing protein may at last be generated.

This is a fundamental change in treatment strategy that promises to render some of the most vexing of today's diseases treatable. Many patients with rare diseases today, like Deepak, if he is still alive, simply don't make an essential protein. That failure to create a single, critical molecule out of the approximately 150,000 protein molecules produced every day by the human body plays out with devastating effect. What's worse is that with a very few exceptions, modern pharmaceuticals today offer nothing more to these patients than they did when I started studying medicine in 1975.

Scientists are making tremendous advances in blocking or camouflaging faulty messages with very precisely targeted new drugs. The work, which has been conducted in animals first, is rapidly maturing. We are now in a position to harness the formidable global resources of science and medicine to find effective and safe treatments for more diseases today than at any previous point in human history.

For families like the Singhs, sadly, it may be too late, but for the next generation of Duchenne boys, we will be close to providing them with highly specific and personal treatment, perhaps at birth, that will allow them to lead full and active lives.

And this revolution won't be limited just to those suffering rare diseases. The shift from an illness to a wellness model, employing information about your genetic makeup to predict subsequent disease and prescribing very precisely targeted medicines, will benefit everyone. Those suffering from common and rare ailments alike.

The genomic information revolution already permits some of today's downstream therapeutics to be used safely with more confidence. That predictive capacity will only grow. The favored approach for developing new drugs even for common diseases will soon be to tackle the faulty messages from mutant genes.

These new technologies will necessitate significant changes in medical education, regulatory review and approval, marketing and reimbursement. These changes are already starting. The U.S. Food and Drug Administration recognizes the need to change. In their October 2011 publication "Driving Biomedical Innovation: Initiatives to Improve Products for Patients," they acknowledge the challenges facing new drugs inherent in the current regulatory pathway, and the need for change to ensure continuing American leadership of global drug development.

As medicine evolves, so too will the physician's work. The next generation of doctors will routinely interpret genomic data and guide you to make lifestyle decisions earlier, including encouraging you to use these highly targeted medications before you develop symptoms. It's an entirely different skills set from those needed now to battle already established disease, which is what doctors are trained for today. Physicians will still need to monitor for early disease, but the effort will become much less invasive, more community-based, and focused especially on you if you are predicted to be at higher risk.

It's even possible that huge hospital facilities will go out of style because the extensive testing and intervention we use them for nowadays will no longer be necessary.

Drug development and regulation will adapt in exciting ways. Currently, the multiple steps of testing necessary for a drug to be proven safe and effective too often rely on a good dose of luck. With science able to more precisely predict how new drugs will work, in whom, when and at what dose, luck will no longer be a principal ingredient of that process. Such precisely targeted medicines might be tested on fewer patients and still be proven safe.

These fundamental changes will lead to alterations in how personalized medicines are manufactured, labeled, distributed, stored, marketed, sold, and reimbursed.

And that will trigger a change in the way society views the role of medicine and doctors.

Currently, you may turn to your physician with a disease already established and their skill at diagnosis and prescribing treatment or performing surgery clearly bears on the outcome. In the future, their most valuable skill will be helping you make wiser lifestyle, behavioral, and medical decisions. The doctor-patient relationship will be different, less paternalistic perhaps, but no less powerful.

And with the benefit of knowledge about your personal genetic makeup, the relationship you have with your physician will become much more personal. After all, your physician will have access to the blueprint that makes you "you."

With this book, I dare to dream about a world where healthcare and lifestyle decisions will one day be taught alongside reading, writing and arithmetic at the heart of education available for all. It will still be up to you whether to follow the advice from your doctor, but in the future the confidence with which that advice is given will be much greater than today. This is truly the greatest leap that medicine has ever made, and with it, medicine will keep us well enough to enjoy a long, happy, and healthy life. For those unlucky enough to have disease-causing genetic mutations, the new era will allow you to truly defy your DNA.

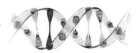

Chapter Two

Medicine through the Millennia

To understand the importance of the latest medical breakthrough, it would be helpful to understand where we come from as human beings, trying to heal ourselves from whatever ails us.

But although it's easy to track the beginning of the current revolution in medicine, when and how did we start ingesting foreign substances to restore our vitality?

The story doesn't start with us humans.

Don't worry; I'm not talking about creatures from outer space.

It started with apes. Not just apes. Primates.

In today's world, local tribesmen have been observed to watch and copy what plants primates eat. Then they use the same plants for the same anti-parasitic reasons. So we humans have been learning from our primate cousins for many millennia. The truth is, animals have an uncanny instinct for knowing the curative properties of plant extracts and making brilliant use of them. Chimpanzees in Africa (Figure 2.1 #1), for instance, routinely seek out and consume plants with antibiotic and antiparasitic properties. They even mix plant extracts and soil rich in the clay mineral, kaolinite, a chemical that improves the potency of the plant extracts. It was also an ingredient in the original version of Kaopectate, until the 1980s. The clay also binds the toxins released by fungi and bacteria that the chimps may have ingested, thus offering protection from potentially harmful foods. Furthermore, kaolin enhances the beneficial effect of the consumed leaves from native plants.

Gorillas in Africa and other primates in South America (Figure 2.1, #1) have also been observed to self-medicate, in some cases consuming poisonous leaves from plants that they normally avoid to cure constipation or protect against gastrointestinal parasites.

But it's not just primates who have an instinct for medicinal products. Elephants trek over dangerous terrain to a cave in Mount Elgon in Kenya to excavate and then grind up particular rocks rich in sodium to counteract toxins found in the plants that they feed on.

Closer to home, you may have noticed your dog or cat chewing on grass to make themselves vomit, expel the grass, and presumably other ingested products which some sense warned them were potentially harmful. So our initial understanding that plants could improve our health initially came from animals.

Then we took the ball and ran with it.

Whatever you think of primitive folk medicine, a lot of it worked. Pharmacologists have now identified active ingredients in poppy (opium), coca (cocaine), foxglove (digitalis), and many more plant extracts all of which were used in primitive folk medicine, and are familiar to doctors even today.

Medicines derived from active plant extracts have been employed by every society from every corner of the globe since ancient times.

The Far East

In ancient China, where acupuncture has been practiced for upward of five thousand years, herbalism has had a similar length of documented use. Recent pottery shards have been found in a Chinese cave dating back twenty thousand years (Figure 2.1, #2). Perhaps these shards were from pots used to store medicinal herbs, as humans moved from hunter-gatherers to settler-farmers?

One of the earliest recorded proponents of herbalism was Emperor Shen Nung who wrote "Pen Ts'ao," or Great Herbal, in ~ 2700 BC describing 365 herbs, many of which it is believed he tested on himself. He is also credited with discovering tea, which acts as an antidote against the poisonous effects of some seventy herbs, which he first tasted in 2737 BC by accident. He was burning tea twigs, with the leaves still on them, when the burning leaves floated up from the fire born by the hot air, landing in his cauldron of boiling water which he subsequently drank. Shen Nung is venerated as the Father of Chinese medicine as well as the first tea drinker.

The Middle East

In Egypt by about two thousand BC, medical prescriptions recorded on papyri were based on plant matter and made reference to the herbalist's combination of medicines and magic for healing. Perhaps the best known of these is the Papyrus Ebers, the most complete and extensive of surviving ancient herbals which dates from 1550 BC (Figure 2.1, #3). The Papyrus Ebers in turn is based on sources, now lost, dating back a further five hundred to two thousand years.

The earliest Sumerian herbal dates from about twenty five hundred BC. In Babylon, many early Arabs were also enthusiasts for herbal remedies. Inscribed Assyrian tablets dated 668–626 BC list about 250 vegetable-based drugs, including many familiar herbs and spices such as saffron, cumin, turmeric and sesame, that are still in use today – and familiar to most cooks.

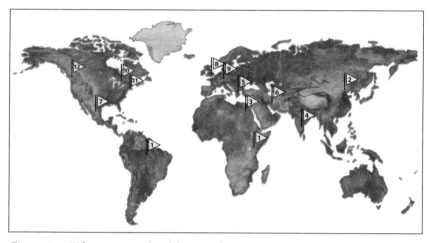

Figure 2.1. Wherever mankind has set foot, so the desire to take medicine to combat disease has followed. See text for flags numbered 1-10. #11 is Harvard University, Boston where Professor Paul Zamecnik first conducted an "antisense experiment." And #12 is Bothell, Washington, the corporate office of my former company, AVI BioPharma (now Sarepta Therapeutics) who have pioneered splice-switching oligomers.

India

Traditional herbal medicine dates back in India at least to the second millennium BC, where it is known as Ayurveda (Figure 2.1, #4). One authentic textbook is the Sushruta Samhita, a book of 184 chapters describing 1,120 illnesses and 821 preparations based on plant, mineral, and animal sources. Sushruta is credited with writing the Sushruta Samhita in Sanskrit, which is a redacted text on all of the major concepts of Ayurvedic medicine with innovative chapters on surgery, then considered the most important branch. Cataract surgery was performed by Sushruta before eight hundred BC.

Europe

From Ancient Greece (Figure 2.1, #5), Hippocrates (460–377 BC) arguably had the greatest influence on modern medicine, and was known to use approximately four hundred different drugs, mostly of plant origin. He is referred to as the father of Western medicine and credited with greatly advancing the systematic study of clinical medicine, summing up the medical knowledge of previous schools.

The First Millennium

Pliny the Elder (Gaius Plinius Secundas, 23-75AD) was a Roman author, naturalist, and natural philosopher. He wrote seven books (as part of a thirty-seven book treatise entitled *Naturalis Historia*) describing medicinal plants that were often cited in other later texts. *Naturalis Historia* became the earliest printed herbal when it was subsequently produced in 1469.

The Islamic World

In the medieval Islamic world, Muslim botanists and physicians made a major contribution to the knowledge of herbal medicines. The most prominent of these is Rhazes (865-925), a Persian physician, alchemist, philosopher, chemist, and scholar. He was the first to differentiate smallpox from measles and discovered kerosene. He has been considered "probably the greatest and most original of all the physicians, and one of the most prolific as an author."

There were many other Persian herbalists, and herbs and chemical compounds were so important that the first known drugstore was opened in Baghdad in 754 AD (Figure 2.1, #6).

The Second Millennium
The Americas

Herbs were also being used in the Americas, by indigenous Aztecs in the South especially. An illustrated herbal published in Mexico in 1552, *Libellus de Medicinalibus Indorum* in the Aztec Nauhuatl language ("Book of Medicinal Herbs of the Indies"), was written by a native physician, Martín de la Cruz (Figure 2.1, #7). The formal illustrations in this book resemble European ones, suggesting that the artist was influenced by his Spanish masters. The book was translated into Latin by Juan Badianus and illustrated the *tlahçolteoçacatl*, *tlayapaloni*, *axocotl*, and *chicomacatl* plants, which were used to make a "remedy for a wounded body" in Aztec herbalism.

Native Americans in North America likely also developed primitive medicines from roots, herbs, and plant extracts but passed the information down through the generations by verbal means rather than written documentation. The healing skills of ancient native peoples have only relatively recently started to be recognized, let alone documented with a written record.

Europe

During the Middle Ages and then the Renaissance, when many sciences progressed considerably in Western Europe, the study and advancement of medicine and drugs did not. Prescriptions generally followed the herbal remedies of ancient cultures, or worse, used bile, animal dung, ground up sexual organs, urine and sweat.

The stimulus for herbalism to become more systematic was the invention of the printing press with a movable typeface, which took place in Germany in 1440. The new printed herbals were more detailed with greater general appeal, often with Gothic script and the addition of woodcut illustrations that more closely resembled the plants being described.

William Turner (1508 to 1568) was an English naturalist, botanist, and theologian who, after studying at Cambridge University, eventually became known as the "father of English botany" (Figure 2.1, #8). He achieved botanical notoriety with his 1538 publication *Libellus de re herbaria novus*, which, despite its title, was the first essay on scientific botany written in English. His three-part *A New Herball* of 1551, 1562, and 1568, was noted for its original contributions and extensive medicinal content and for being written in vernacular English. The woodcut illustrations he included however were taken from an earlier work by the German botanist, Leonhart Fuchs (1501-1566). Turner described over two hundred species of plants native to England and his work had a strong influence on later eminent botanists such as John Ray and Jean Bauhin.

John Gerard (1545–1612) was the most popular of the English herbalists due to his publication, in 1596, of *Catalogus*. This was a list of 1033 plants growing in his Elizabethan English garden at Holborn, where he introduced exotic plants from the New World. In 1597, he published the large and heavily illustrated *Herball, or Generall Historie of Plantes*, which went on to be the most widely circulated botany book in English in the seventeenth century.

In the seventeenth century, greater interest in medicine in England was stimulated by the English physician, Thomas Sydenham (1624-1689). Sydenham fought for the Parliamentarians under Oliver Cromwell throughout the English Civil War, and, at its end, resumed his medical studies at Magdalene College, Oxford. He published widely on medical topics and gave the needed boost to pharmacology and was posthumously accorded the title of "English Hippocrates." Among Sydenham's many achievements was the discovery of a disease, Sydenham's Chorea, also known as St. Vitus Dance. This is a disease of characteristic jerky movements of the limbs and grimacing of the facial muscles, often occurring in children and caused by an infection with the *Streptococcus* bacterium that was often associated with rheumatic heart fever.

John Parkinson (1567–1650), a founding member of the Worshipful Society of Apothecaries, was apothecary to King James I of England, who was also King James VI of Scotland. Parkinson was an enthusiastic and skillful gardener, stocking his garden in Long Acre, in Covent Garden, London, with many rare plants. Parkinson was the last of the great English herbalists and one of the first of the great English botanists.

Parkinson was an active correspondent with important English and Continental herbalists and botanists, and imported many new and unusual plants from overseas, in particular from the Mediterranean coast of the Middle East and from Virginia on the U.S. East Coast. Parkinson is celebrated for his two monumental works, the first *Paradisi in Sole Paradisus Terrestris* in 1629. This was essentially a gardening book for which Charles I awarded him the title Royal Botanist. The second was his *Theatrum Botanicum* or Theatre of Plants, of 1640. This was the largest herbal ever produced in the English language and was the most complete and beautifully-presented treatise on plants of its time.

Another British example from the period is the astrologically-themed *Complete Herbal* written in 1653 by the physician and astrologer Nicholas Culpeper (1616-1654), based on his experience cataloging English herbs. Culpeper's book was reprinted many times and remained popular with many even into the twentieth century. However, by including astrological themes the book never gained scientific authority and credibility with all physicians then or since.

Culpepper, a radical republican, fought for Cromwell during the English Civil War and performed heroic surgery while battles raged about him. Culpeper was no friend of the medical establishment at the time, believing physicians overcharged for their services and by not publishing work, or publishing in Latin, were deliberately trying to keep their patients in ignorance. So while many were preoccupied with the war he set about publishing his work in vernacular English, outraging the Royal College of Physicians. He also charged little for his printed leaflets further upsetting his professional brethren. Culpepper's main work, *The English Physician*, was published in 1708 in Boston. It became the most successful non-religious English text of all time, with many readers in colonial America, and remains in print today at $35 for the 94 page hardback edition.

However, despite the efforts of such enlightened physician herbalists as Sydenham, Parkinson, and Culpeper in both Britain and mainland Europe, treatment of illness often involved administering poisons, bleeding or "cupping" and application of clysters, what we know as enemas, purges and sudorifics to increase sweating. Today, nobody would be surprised at the lack of efficacy of these barbaric measures, which did little to endear physicians to their gullible patients.

In the nineteenth century, there were efforts to identify, isolate and purify the medicinal extracts from plants. Friedrich Serturner (1783-1841), a German pharmacist, was the first to isolate any plant extract, an alkaloid from the poppy plant in 1804. He found the extract induced dream-like states in people, so he named the extract morphium after Morpheus, the Greek god of dreams. Serturner subsequently purified the extract and marketed it as morphine, from his pharmacy in Einbeck in 1817 (Figure 2.1, #9).

An Italian chemist, Raffaele Piria (1814 – 1865) isolated and prepared salicyclic acid from salicin – originally from willow trees. Later, in 1853, a French chemist, Charles Gerhardt (1816-1856) synthesized the derivative acetylsalicylic acid, with later refinements to the process by Karl-Johann Kraut in 1869 and Hermann Kolbe in 1874. It wasn't until 1899 when the German company, Bayer, introduced the compound as aspirin that it became the first fever reducing, widely marketed, pure drug.

The 20th Century

The development of drugs became an established science in 1909 when Paul Ehrlich (1854-1915), a Prussian Jew, discovered an arsenic-based drug, called Salvarsan, to treat syphilis. Ehrlich was awarded the Nobel Prize for Physiology or Medicine for his work on infectious disease and Salvarsan became the best selling drug in the world between 1910 and the 1940s when it was eventually replaced by penicillin.

These early drugs were developed by a chemical synthetic process, in test tubes on a small scale and in big vats on a larger scale. Soon, drugs would be created by biological processes using living cells. Yeasts or bacteria were initially used to produce the product. More recently, biological drugs have been produced in tissue cultures. The biologic products are generally much bigger molecules, often complex, and can be protein, sugar, nucleic acid or a combination of these. If the biologic is a protein made by cells from an animal, it may create an allergic reaction to the foreign animal protein once given to humans.

The first biologic drug was insulin, which was first isolated by Frederick Banting and Charles Best in Toronto in the 1920s (Figure 2.1, #10). That was followed by cortisone, isolated by Edward Kendall at the Mayo Clinic in Rochester, Minnesota. Kendall won a Nobel Prize in 1950. Thereafter small molecule drugs, and to a lesser extent biologics, began to establish a greater potential place in medicine. By the early twentieth century, modern pharmaceuticals had arrived, less than one hundred years ago.

The First Biologic Drug

Dr. Frederick Banting and Charles Best, then a medical student, conducted experiments with insulin in dogs who had had their

---

pancreas removed, to make them diabetic. Pancreatic extract was injected into a diabetic dog in the summer of 1921. The dog's elevated blood glucose level dropped, and it seemed healthier and stronger. The intrepid duo kept their diabetic dog in healthy condition by injecting it with the extract several times a day. In late 1921, biochemist Bertram Collip joined the team that was now tasked with purifying the insulin extracted from the pancreas of cattle so that it would be clean enough for testing on humans. In January 1922, in Toronto, a 14-year-old boy was the first human diabetic to receive insulin. Before the insulin shots he was near death. But the test was a success and he rapidly regained his strength and appetite. Soon, Eli Lilly started large-scale production of the extract and by 1923 was producing enough insulin to supply the entire North American continent.

Drugs aimed at specific targets, which are the direct antecedents to medicines that target genes, began to emerge in 1935 with Sulfanilamide. This was an antibacterial drug discovered by Gerhard Domagk (another Nobel laureate) and Therese Trefouel. It was in all likelihood the first drug that reacted with a specific protein receptor. Then in 1940, Thaddeus Mann and David Keilin in Cambridge, UK, discovered that sulfanilamide encouraged urinary excretion by blocking the enzyme carbonic anhydrase, thus working as a diuretic as well as an antibiotic.

This led to the successful search for more potent carbonic anhydrase inhibitors, which act to reduce elevated blood pressure and are called anti-hypertensives.

Other small molecules began to be sought in order to target other specific protein receptors.

The Placebo Effect

In 1955, it was discovered that if a patient believed in a substance, it could create a healing effect even if it had no actual pharmacological value. Henry Beecher wrote about the "*Powerful Placebo*" in the Journal of the American Medical Association. He noted that a dummy drug, the placebo, worked in about a third of cases. This was true even when it was prescribed by a physician. And it was true for a range of diseases too, from an upper respiratory infection to a headache.

Given the wide diversity of patients treated with any one pharmacologically active compound, the diversity of responses, and our still limited knowledge about how drugs work in some cases, a response rate of 33% is not very different from the response rate seen with some drugs. Thus, over the last fifty years, and especially recently, drugs are compared with the placebo effect when evaluating how effective they are. That is not to say that the drug's mechanism of action is unknown or incorrect. It is just that the interaction between disease and patient is far more complex than was previously thought.

Once a potential drug has been identified, then making it, purifying it and ensuring its stability can commence. Testing in the laboratory, so called *in vitro* testing, to see if the drug does indeed interact with the target receptor, is the next step. These target receptors are often obtained in a blood test or biopsy from a patient with the disease in question. This *in vitro* work takes place prior to any work being conducted in whole animals, called *in vivo* work.

By now the potential drug is called a New Chemical Entity, NCE or New Molecular Entity, NME. Confirming that this potential drug does indeed interact with the target can be a lengthy process, called

Proof of Principle. Once convincing proof has been obtained in the laboratory which is another complex process, preliminary safety testing in animals can start.

It was hoped that modern technology and knowledge would alleviate the need to test NCEs in animals (see Chapter 9); however, that hope has not been realized yet. That is despite computerization and the greater understanding about the various drug classes, chemical subgroups and modifications and their predictable effects, that nowadays go into building an NCE.

The process of discovering, developing and licensing medicinal drugs has become much more complex and costly. This trend is likely to continue, with animal testing remaining an integral and gatekeeping part of that process before any testing in humans is allowed. The regulatory hurdles for NCEs get higher because the public expects new drugs to be marketed that are effective but represent zero risk of adverse effects. This is currently impossible to guarantee, but what is seemingly expected. Attorneys line up to sue any company unlucky enough to market a drug that subsequently is shown be unsafe even in a tiny proportion of patients treated.

Penicillin, the first of the wonder antibiotics, was discovered by Sir Alexander Fleming (1881-1955) in 1928. Fleming, a Scottish biologist and pharmacologist, wrote many articles on bacteriology, immunology, and chemotherapy. He discovered the enzyme lysozyme in 1923. He was a brilliant researcher who fortunately kept an extremely messy laboratory. In August 1928 he stacked all his cultures of the staphylococcus bacteria on a bench in a corner of his laboratory before going on vacation with his family. On returning, on 3rd September, Fleming noticed that one culture was contaminated with a mold that had killed the colonies of staphylococci that immediately surrounded it. Other colonies farther away were normal.

Fleming grew the mold in a pure culture and found that it produced a bacteria-killing substance. He identified the mold as being from the Penicillium genus, and, named the substance it released "penicillin."

Penicillin had to wait for better synthetic manufacturing processes before it could be widely distributed. It initially reached U.S. servicemen in 1941, and then the general public after World War II ended in 1945.

Interestingly enough, it is likely that penicillin had been used for centuries beforehand with the ancient Egyptian practice of using poultices of moldy bread.

Penicillin heralded the "New Age of Antimicrobials," but there has always been one problem with the entire drug category. As fast as new classes of antibiotics have been developed, the microbes against which they are pitted evolve to become resistant to them.

Other major classes of drugs were serendipitously discovered or scientifically developed based on better disease understanding. These advances include the first beta-blocker, propranolol, created by Sir James Black in 1962. Black's work built on the discovery of the adreno-receptor by George Oliver and Edward Schafer at University College, London who showed that adrenal extract, when injected, would raise blood pressure. The active ingredient, adrenaline was discovered in 1904. However the actual molecular target of adrenaline, called epinephrine in the U.S., was only demonstrated to be two classes of protein receptors in 1948, so called alpha and beta receptors. More about the beta receptor, a G-protein coupled receptor, in Chapter 4. Black went to work for ICI Pharmaceuticals in 1958 and it was while there that he developed propranolol, for the treatment of high blood pressure and heart disease.

Other new drug classes, developed in the late twentieth century, based on better disease understanding, include:

- antimigraine triptan drugs to block the 5-hydroxytryptamine receptor
- histamine H_2 receptor antagonists to reduce stomach acid
- proton pump inhibitors to reduce stomach acid
- selective serotonin receptor antagonists to combat depression

By the end of the twentieth century, medicines were classified into Anatomical Therapeutic Chemical (ATC) classes according to what body system they acted on and/or their therapeutic or chemical characteristic. The classification system is "owned" by the World Health Organization Collaborating Centre who established the 14 main ATC groups and they have published updates since the first edition that appeared only as recently as 1976.

Third Millennium

By the end of the first decade in the twenty-first century, there is information available on over thirty thousand medicines that can be prescribed or purchased over the counter. But, as mentioned previously, there are approximately 150,000 proteins in the body, so only a small fraction of these have successfully been targeted by the drugs developed so far. And many of these thirty thousand drugs have been developed by modification of an existing drug and share the same target. More than twenty-five thousand of these drugs have been available for many years and are now off patent. As new targets and small molecule drugs to target them are getting harder to find, some people fear that we are reaching the limit of what is druggable.

Moving into the second decade of this millennium, more research and developmental effort is being focused on the rare diseases that until very recently were considered to be untreatable. Members of the Pharmaceutical Research and Manufacturers of America, America's biopharmaceutical organization, invested an estimated $45.8 billion in 2009 to discover and develop new medicines. Much of this money is being spent on rare diseases, which are both devastating to patients and complex for researchers. By early 2011, a record 460 medicines for rare diseases were in late stages of the drug development pipeline, either in clinical trials or awaiting U.S. Food and Drug Administration (FDA) review.

A rare disease is defined by the U.S. government as one that afflicts fewer than two-hundred thousand Americans. There are approximately seven thousand rare diseases. Half of these afflict children. Eighty percent of these rare diseases affect fewer than six thousand U.S. patients. However, in total, approximately thirty million Americans suffer from one rare disease or another, that's one in every ten of us.

Taken together, rare diseases are common. Across the world, as many as six hundred million patients now suffer from a rare disease. Often, patients suffer from untreatable diseases for years before getting a correct diagnosis. Then they get the news that there is very little or nothing that modern science and medicine can do to help them. However, as this book will demonstrate, there is now hope for some of these six hundred million suffering patients, or at least the next generation of patients who are destined to suffer like them.

The Future of Conventional Drugs

What's the future of conventional drugs in the twenty first century?

In the last thirty years, blockbuster drugs have come and gone. Many have enjoyed enormous peak sales, reflecting their efficacy or benefit and safety. That has provided for a favorable benefit-risk ratio and popularity. The sales have rewarded the marketing machines of the companies that manufactured them. A list of the top twenty drugs by sales is given in Appendix A. Drug marketing has become big business with significant amounts spent on advertising to the medical profession, and in some countries such as the U.S., to the general public as well.

One of the most recognizable of these blockbuster drugs is Ventolin for treating the bronchospasm of asthma. Ventolin is also known by its active chemical name, albuterol in the U.S. or salbutamol in the rest of the world. Ventolin was the first stimulator of the adrenergic beta receptor. It was launched in 1968 by Allen & Hanburys.

Allen & Hanburys is the oldest pharmaceutical company, established in London in 1715. It is now part of the GlaxoSmithKline family. Allen & Hanburys was the company I joined from UK family practice in 1993. So I regard it as my industrial alma mater, as well as Glaxo in general, and I am more familiar with the stories about their blockbuster drugs.

The active ingredient in Ventolin, albuterol/salbutamol, has remained the most frequently prescribed inhaled asthma-reliever medication for approximately 45 years. The patent has long since expired on the salbutamol/albuterol molecule but with Ventolin inhaler having to be reformulated with HFA (hydrofluoroalkane), a different propellant, into a CFC-free (chlorofluorocarbon) inhaler, the brand is once again protected from generic alternative competition until 2015. The new propellant was required to reduce the harm done to the protective ozone layer in our atmosphere by the older CFC propellants. The HFA propellants also have less global warming potential than the older CFC ones. Ventolin is the asthma reliever medication that you may still reach for when you feel your chest go tight or you start wheezing.

Stomach ulcers and excessive stomach acid were at one time treated with cimetidine, a drug used to block the stomach acid-producing histamine H_2 receptor, developed by James Black. Black then refined cimetidine, and in doing so developed another of Glaxo's blockbuster drugs, ranitidine (Zantac), that had fewer adverse drug reactions, was longer-lasting in action, and had ten times more activity than cimetidine. Black was awarded the Nobel Prize for Medicine in 1988 for work leading to the development of propranolol and cimetidine.

Zantac was initially launched in 1981 and by 1988 was the top selling prescription drug in the U.S. It has now become available "Over the Counter" (OTC) in many countries as the long and large safety database established suggests its use no longer needs to be overseen by a physician. The patent on the drug ranitidine expired in 1997 and many generic manufacturers rushed their versions of ranitidine on to the market to capitalize on its popularity, while new classes of drugs, such as the proton pump inhibitors or PPIs were developed and found to be even more effective in treating excessive gastric acid.

Prozac, fluoxetine is the generic name, is another blockbuster drug, developed by Eli Lilly as a selective serotonin reuptake inhibitor, or SSRI. It is perhaps the best known SSRI used for treating major depression, but it was only the fourth to reach the market. Two of the first three SSRIs, zimeldine, indalpine and fluvoxamine, had to be withdrawn because of adverse side effects. Prozac became available in the U.S. in 1987 and became a major blockbuster and the subject of the book "Prozac Nation" by Elizabeth Wurtzel published in 1994, as well as a subsequent film, before its patent too expired in 2001.

Summary

For 4,900 of the last five thousand years, mankind has been limited mostly to using herbs and plants for medicinal purposes.

As science has evolved and brought greater understanding to disease, especially over the last half century, so have new synthetic or natural chemicals been discovered and developed. More recently, biological products have arrived. Both classes have had the goal of "correct or cure", and the science of drug development has exploded onto the scene.

Drugs can be broadly characterized into falling into one of three "platform technologies":

- Small molecules, which can nevertheless be very large
- Biological products, first developed under a hundred years ago
- The "Nucleic acid-based-therapeutics", in the last thirty years.

The dividing line between these platforms is occasionally blurred, but the remainder of this book will focus on the Nucleic acid based-therapeutics which will eventually become established as a major breakthrough for medical science and a source of many new medicines.

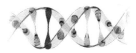

Chapter Three

From Primordial Soup to Personalized Medicine

The building blocks of life on earth began in the hot reactive stew of hydrogen, carbon, oxygen and nitrogen that defined our planet roughly three and a half billion years ago. That was a mere ten billion years after the universe was formed by the Big Bang, and one billion years after our planet had formed. It is there that the rules governing genetics and personalized medicine spawned.

Yet it was only during the last one hundred years that scientists concluded that DNA was the source of genetic inheritance.

Genes and DNA

Think of genes as library books; stacked on shelves (the chromosomes); in a library (the nucleus) of a city (the cell). All free living organisms contain genes, from bacteria to the simplest algae and plants, right up the vegetable and animal kingdoms to us, *homo sapiens*, at the self-proclaimed top of the evolutionary tree. Even viruses, which are not really alive and can only reproduce and manufacture their proteins inside the host cell, require at least a few genes composed of either DNA or RNA.

So what exactly is DNA, deoxyribonucleic acid? It's a polymer, which is a long chain of connected units like the teeth of a zipper, or a string of beads on a necklace. DNA was discovered by Friedrich Miescher, a Swiss physician, in the 1860s. He obtained cells from the pus from discarded surgical bandages, and isolated their nuclei and the material within. He called this nuclear material nucleic acid. Each unit of DNA contains a sugar molecule called deoxyribose. Deoxyribose consists of five atoms. Four carbon atoms and one oxygen in a ring which bind one of the four nucleic acid bases, adenine (A), guanine (G), cytosine (C) or thymine (T). Each [sugar + base unit] is called a nucleoside. The nucleosides are joined to each other by a link, a phosphate group, forming long threads of hundreds of thousands of subunits. These subunits, [sugar + base + phosphate link], are called nucleotides.

RNA is essentially the same as DNA except that it has another oxygen atom included in each ribose sugar molecule. So a DNA sugar unit is actually an RNA sugar unit without one oxygen, which is why it has the name "deoxy-ribose."

Miescher thought nucleic acid could only have a simple and boring function, since DNA molecules are composed of long strings of nucleotides that are almost identical apart from having one of four possible bases attached. He thought that it might serve as a kind of scaffolding that just sat in the nucleus and supported more "interesting" molecules such as proteins. Proteins in turn are made up of strings of amino acids, of which there are twenty-two different varieties.

Nothing could be further from the truth!

On each ribose, or deoxyribose, unit another chemical is added. In the case of DNA these are one of the four bases: adenosine (A), guanine

(G), cytosine (C) and thymine (T). When James Watson and Francis Crick elucidated the double helix crystal structure of DNA in 1953, they found that these four bases "partner up."

The Unknown Heroine Behind Watson and Crick

Rosalind Franklin (1920 – 1958) was a British biophysicist, and graduate of Cambridge University, who used X-rays while working at the Medical Research Council Biophysics Unit at King's College, London to define crystal structures. It was her data on the structure of DNA, and in particular photograph 51, that Watson and Crick relied on, without her knowledge, or much recognition, to work out the structure of DNA. Her articles, which outlined the structure of DNA based on her own work, were eventually published in the same issue of *Nature* as Watson and Crick's better known paper. Franklin, Crick, Watson and Maurice Wilkins were keen to beat Linus Pauling to establish the actual structure of DNA after Pauling had proposed an incorrect structure for DNA.

When the four bases "partner up", they are bound, weakly, by hydrogen bonds: A binds to T and vice versa; C binds to G, and again vice versa. Adenine and guanine are examples of purine bases, and cytosine and thymine are pyrimidines (Figure 3.1a). In DNA, a long strand of the linked deoxyribose sugars bearing one of the four bases on each sugar molecule, now called deoxyribonucleic acid, is "zipped up" by pairing with a complementary chain of nucleotides (Figure 3.1b) on the other DNA strand. These long paired chains of complementary nucleotides (i.e. double strands) are then wound into a helix (Figure 3.1c), folded and balled up, to make up genes, which in turn are linked together on chromosomes.

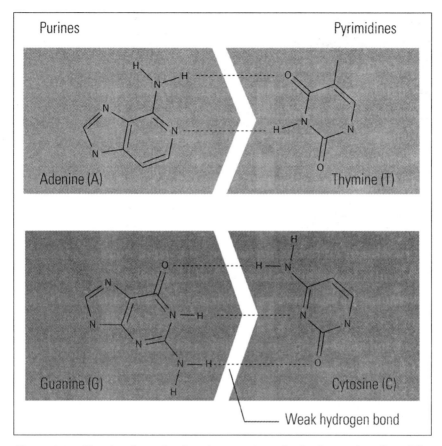

Purines   Pyrimidines

Adenine (A)   Thymine (T)

Guanine (G)   Cytosine (C)

———— Weak hydrogen bond

Figure 3.1a. Showing how the four bases pair up by hydrogen bonding. The pyrimidine base Thymine (T) partners with the purine base, Adenine (A), and the pyrimidine base, Cytosine (C) partners up with the purine base Guanine (G). These bases are then attached to the deoxyribose sugar rings of DNA or the ribose sugar rings of RNA. The sugars are joined together by phosphate linkages to form phosphate-deoxyribose or phosphate-ribose backbones accordingly (Figure 3.1b). Each deoxyribose plus base plus phosphate unit is called a nucleotide. The nucleotides are joined together into very long sequences, often over a million units long. In the case of DNA these then line up against their complementary partners to form a double strand, and are then wound into the characteristic double helix formation (Figure 3.1c)

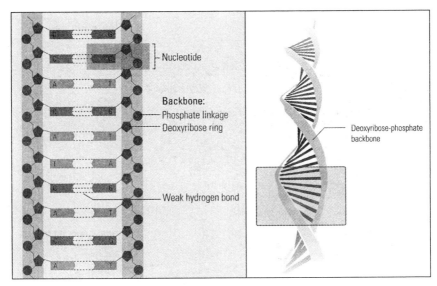

Figure 3.1b. The phosphate-deoxyribose backbone of DNA.

Figure 3.1c. The characteristic double strand formation of DNA, wound into a double helix, which is then further folded and twisted.

DNA is a great way to store and transmit information, in this case, genetic information. But more than that, scientists have even been able to store information in strands of DNA that you or I would think more likely belong on a computer. Recently, a team led by Professor George Church at Harvard, reported in the magazine, *Science*, that they had stored a 53,000 word book, including eleven images and a computer program (5.27 megabits of information), in a strand of DNA. The scientists went on to suggest that as the technology improves we might see DNA replacing conventional computers. One gram of DNA, about the weight of a pinch of salt, can store 455 billion gigabytes of information. That is the same amount of information that today would be stored on one hundred billion DVDs!

There are advantages of storing information in DNA, as all species on this planet have found. It is easily copied and passed on to the next generation. It can still be read thousands of years later, as we are now doing with the DNA from Egyptian mummies. And the way to read DNA does not change, unlike the rapidly changing digital storage media that make today's information technology breakthroughs tomorrow's relics for the museum or recycling.

Chromosomes

We humans have 46 chromosomes, consisting of 22 pairs and two sex chromosomes (XX in the case of women and XY in the case of men) (Figure 3.2). On these chromosomes, we have approximately 25,000 genes in total.

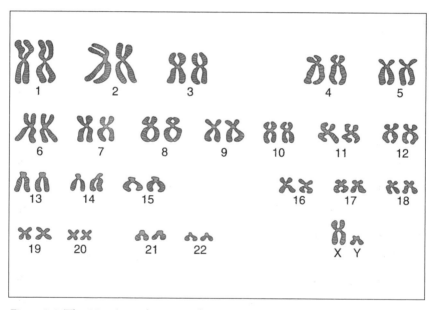

Figure 3.2. The 22 pairs and two sex chromosomes (in this case from a man – with the characteristic, short Y sex chromosome) of a human.

Most of our genes regulate the production of a protein of some description, with different genes in different parts of the body being more active than elsewhere. Think of it as the information, the blueprint, in the books (genes) being taken out of the library and sent to a house or factory (the ribosome). The ribosomes are small organelles within the same city, the cell, where this information can then be read, understood and used to produce something – in this case a protein. The ribosome is a protein-making machine in the outer part of the cell.

Each and every nucleated cell in the body has the same library, with the same 25,000 books, the genes. But different types of cells will be programmed to produce different proteins by taking the information from different books in the library. The book, in this case the gene, does not leave the library, the nucleus, but the information, the blueprint it contains, is conveyed to the ribosome factory in the cell cytoplasm by a messenger, a copy of the information. That copy is messenger RNA, mRNA.

RNA

Messenger RNA is cleverly made. When the double strand of DNA in the nucleus unzips, new sequences of complementary material bind to the exposed single strand of DNA and are then peeled off (transcribed) as precursor messenger RNA (pre-mRNA) (Figure 3.3). In the process, RNA incorporates the pyrimidine base Uracil (U) instead of the Thymine that is found in DNA. The formed RNA units [ribose+base+phosphate linkage] are also called nucleotides.

However, there is much information within these DNA strands that is currently considered unnecessary. Think of the "book" (the gene) being composed of many chapters. In the case of the largest gene in the body, that for dystrophin, the gene consists of 2,400,000,000 nucleotide units. These nucleotides are split up into "sections" (chapters) of exons and introns. For dystrophin, there are 79 exons (accounting for 0.6% of the gene's sequence) and 78 introns (accounting for the remaining 99.4% of the 2.4 billion letters of the gene). Only the exons are needed for the information they contain to be translated into the dystrophin protein by the ribosome. Most of dystrophin's exons are relatively small at between 23 and 269 nucleotides in length, compared to the average size of the dystrophin introns, which are over 26,000 nucleotides long.

All the information required by the muscle cell for manufacturing the final protein, dystrophin, is contained in the 79 exons – just 0.6% of the dystrophin gene.

Figure 3.3. Simple diagram of transcription initiation. RNA polymerase is an enzyme that unzips the double strand of DNA, and moves down the gene (black coding thread).

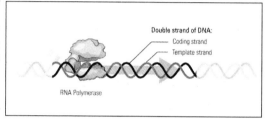

As the double strand "unzips" the polymerase assembles complementary RNA units which gradually lengthen as the gene unzips, and then zips back up again.

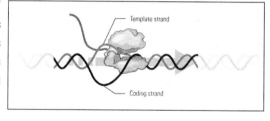

Eventually, the gene has generated a full complementary RNA strand and transcription terminates. The new pre messenger RNA is completed and released. The DNA double strand "zips" back up, and the RNA polymerase is free to work on another gene.

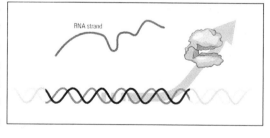

The introns, by and large, carry information that is not needed by the factory in the cell cytoplasm, so they can be removed as the pre-mRNA is tidied up and converted into useful mRNA. We now know that this process of "tidying up", which is called splicing, is a complex process, performed in the nucleus, and may in fact lead to different, "alternative", blueprints being sent to the different cellular factories.

The Encyclopedia of DNA Elements (ENCODE) consortium of 442 researchers, launched by the U.S. National Human Genome Research Institute in 2003, has been examining the 99% of DNA that make up the introns. In September 2012, the scientists published 30 papers simultaneously in three major scientific journals, a remarkable feat on its own. In those papers many common diseases such as diabetes, obesity, heart disease, cancer and Alzheimer's dementia, the ones that are not caused by identified single genes, are now thought to be caused by genes being switched on or off by the information contained in the introns. But the story is only just beginning to be unraveled. We have a long way to go to fully understand what 99% of our DNA does, and how. A whole new branch of medicine and range of possible new drugs is now emerging that will target these switches that may trigger a liver cell to stop absorbing sugar and so diabetes develops; or the switch which once thrown in a lung cell will turn it into a cancer cell.

It used to be thought that one gene codes for one protein, but we now know that there are roughly 25,000 genes but approximately 150,000 proteins. Thus each gene on average contains the blueprint for six proteins. How?

The process of tidying up can sometimes lead to the message (in mRNA) being put together in different ways. Imagine that the book in the library is taken off the shelf and the cover and binding are removed, the non-essential information (the introns) is discarded (more about that later) and then a copy of the necessary information is bound into a much, much slimmer book. Thus the book copy (mRNA) that will leave the library (nucleus) only contains important instructions so that when it reaches the factory (the ribosome in the cell cytoplasm), the various blueprints are still recognized and can still be used to build the finished products (the different proteins). The introns that have been discarded contained no useful information at all, or so it was thought, but all of the exons do contain useful information. However sometimes one exon, or more, is missing from the final mRNA that makes it to the ribosome and some of the useful instruction is missing. A different final protein product can still sometimes be made and may work for the cell, and the body.

If the "book copy" (mRNA) was the blueprint for a car (protein), then consider that there would be chapters (exons) on how many wheels it had as well as a chapter on how many seats it had. It would have a chapter on the interior finish, another on the size of the engine, what color it should be, where and how the alarm is set up, etc. All of these chapters would be necessary to produce the car as sold in the showroom functioning to the manufacturer's specifications. However, if the chapter on the alarm was missing, the car would still work; it just wouldn't have an alarm. Or the car might be a different color, or lack one or more coats of paint. The car might rust quicker, but it would still be drivable.

Thus 25,000 genes (books in the library), may each generate many different molecules of mRNA (copies of thinned down books consisting of important information - exons). On average each gene in our bodies generates six different mRNA molecules that leave the library (nucleus) and go to the factory (ribosome), where they will generate six times the number of proteins compared to the number of original genes. This process, first described in 1977, is called alternative splicing.

Alternative splicing

We now know that 95% of our genes, those that are composed of multiple exons, are alternatively spliced. This happens across all eukaryote species. Eukaryote species are plants and animals where the cell has a nucleus and other discrete structures, as opposed to prokaryotes, bacteria, where the cells do not have these discrete structures. The current record for most mRNA variants being generated from a single gene comes from the fruit fly, *Drosophila melanogaster.* The humble fruit fly has a gene, *Dscam,* which generates more than 38,000 splice variants.

The fruit fly has long been used to study genetics. In this interesting insect, alternative splicing is required to produce offspring of each gender. Pre-mRNAs from the *D. melanogaster* gene *dsx* contain 6 exons. In males, exons 1, 2, 3, 5, and 6 (skipping exon 4) are joined to form the mRNA, which codes for a regulatory protein required for male development. In females, exons 1, 2, 3, and 4 are joined (leaving out exons 5 and 6). The resulting mRNA is a regulatory protein required for female development. (Also see Figure 4.1).

Continuing the analogy of the book (or blueprint) ending up at the factory (ribosome) out in the cell cytoplasm (the city). The book is composed of words. Each word is composed of three letters but the words all make sense. Each letter is a nucleotide and each word (of three nucleotides) is a codon. Codons are bundled together – sometimes only a few, other times thousands, to form chapters in the book. Each chapter is an exon. The blueprint makes sense if the words in a chapter make sense. However, sometimes the book is damaged and a chapter, several words, or even a single letter in a word, is missing. The process of tidying up the book into a manageable copy "splices" the chapters of useful information (exons) together and removes the non-essential information (introns), by arranging every word (codon) with three letters (nucleotides) into sentences. The mRNA strand (the copy of the blueprint) can then be translated by the factory (the ribosome) into a protein.

However, if a single letter is missing, during the transcription process a letter is taken from the next word to complete the previous word. The factory can only read words in sequence. Each word has to be of three letters during this "splicing" for the sentence (and hence the chapter, and thus the book) to make sense. If the words are spliced incorrectly, the book cannot be "read", and the factory (ribosome) will not be able to make the protein.

Consider this example:

> ➤ *the big red fox ran far and saw the dog and cat hit the man*

This information can be read and understood, but if the "g" is missed in big, then "r" is used from red to complete the codon, frame shift occurs and the sentence no longer makes any sense:

> ➤ *the bir edf oxr anf ara nds awt hed oga ndc ath itt hem an*

In practice, the factory will start off reading the message. It will be able to follow the instructions for "the," but none of the other codons will make sense. So the rest of the sentence will not be interpreted, or worse, may generate bad proteins. This situation occurs in some, perhaps many, rare genetically determined diseases. It is estimated that 70% of neurological diseases are associated with some form of upset in the regulation of alternative splicing.

There are 64 possible codons of three letters generated by the four bases A, C, G and T. Any one of the four bases can be placed in any of the three positions in the codon, thus the number of possible options is 4 x 4 x 4, which equals 64.

Protein is composed of chains of amino acids. There are 21 amino acids of which twenty are coded for by one or more of the 64 individual possible codons. That is why it is vital for the three letters in a codon to be faithfully reproduced. If a different sequence of three letters is made, either no amino acid will be coded for, or the wrong one is included. This may turn the protein from a "good" protein into a "bad" protein as in the case of sickle cell anemia, where a single nucleotide mutation leads to the hydrophobic (water hating) amino acid valine replacing the hydrophilic (water loving) amino acid glutamic acid on one of the hemoglobin protein chains.

Sickle Cell Anemia

Sickle cell anemia is prevalent in the tropics and especially in sub-Saharan Africa where roughly one third of indigenous people carry the recessive gene. In Africa, carrying one copy of the gene (as it is recessive, the disease only occurs if both parents contribute one copy of the sickle gene), has over the centuries provided some protection against malaria, providing a compensatory benefit. This survival advantage has allowed this otherwise unhealthy trait to remain widely prevalent in Africa where malaria too is prevalent.

Those unlucky enough to be homozygous and to have two copies of the sickle gene find their red blood cells become rigid and distorted under the microscope, acquiring the characteristic sickle shape, and they get stuck in the small capillaries robbing downstream tissue of oxygen getting destroyed in the process, leading to anemia.

Healthy red blood cells generally survive 90 to 120 days before being replaced, but sickle cells only last 10 to 20 days, and the bone marrow cannot keep pace with this rapid turnover. In 1956, Vernon Ingram

---

45

(1924 – 2006), a professor of biology at the Massachusetts Institute of Technology, along with John Hunt and Antony Stretton, first reported that sickle cell anemia was caused by a single amino acid substitution in the hemoglobin molecule. This led to Ingram being credited as the "Father of Molecular Medicine".

Summary

The city (cell) has a library (nucleus) containing 46 shelves (chromosomes) of books (genes) made of original paper (DNA). Each book (gene) in the library contains many chapters of useful information (exons) and unnecessary information (introns – or at least we currently believe that most introns do not provide useful information). Each chapter (exon) is composed of many words (codons) of three letters (nucleotides). The factory in the cell does not need the original book from the library – just a copy of the useful information (contained in the exons) from the book. At the shelves, the book is taken to pieces and the original codons of 3 letters (A, T, C, and G) matched up with complementary letters (U, A, G and C) of a growing strand of precursor mRNA. This whole copy of the book, as pre-mRNA, is sent to be rebound ("spliced") by the librarian (the "spliceosome"), where the non-essential information is discarded and the remaining chapters are "rebound" as the mature mRNA, which then leaves the library and heads to the factory. I have tried to simplify this complex process while describing, with some license, the main steps. Each year, more is understood about the process, the various signaling and regulating chemicals and even more questions arise.

How does the spliceosome form and why? Somewhere, someone is beavering away on that very question.

What controls the rate at which these processes progress, the rebinding for instance?

What controls the rate at which the books are taken off the shelves?

How is the speed at which the newly bound books leave the library regulated?

Intense investigation is trying to reveal the mechanisms that perform these important controls.

We do know now that there are other types of RNA, microRNA and regulatory RNA, which seem to control some of these steps. The introns, previously thought to contain no vital information, may be critical and involved in these processes. As science phrases the important questions and the answers are discovered, correcting misconceptions, new questions will be raised.

Right now, we are already beginning to develop synthetic oligomers which will camouflage small pieces of the messenger RNA in some cases triggering alternative splicing, and thus giving us medicines to defy some of our previously untreatable diseases.

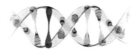

Chapter Four

Camouflage Your Genes

The drugs we use today interfere with disease processes once they have started, instead of getting to the root of the problem.

In the future, though, doctors will be able to prescribe medicines earlier in a disease process, even before symptoms develop. This will be accomplished by more precisely targeting drugs, based on genetics, to smaller numbers of people with a specific set of genes, or a single mutated gene.

Doctors armed with genetic information will be more confident that the benefits of these therapies outweigh harm for a specific patient. They'll also know when to avoid their use altogether in those patients who are genetically most likely to experience side effects.

Indeed, we have already identified some of these genes that make certain drugs safe for many, but dangerous for a few. Consider again the case of Coumadin (warfarin) discussed in Chapter One. Doctors frequently prescribe warfarin for atrial fibrillation (AF), a common condition affecting millions of Americans in their forties and fifties. AF causes one of the upper two chambers (atria) of the heart to "flutter" or fail to contract regularly, or effectively enough to push blood through the heart, into the lungs and back, and then out to the rest of the body. People with AF end up feeling breathless and fatigued. In addition, blood can pool in the ineffective atrium and clot. These clots may then dislodge and travel to the brain where they cause strokes, or travel to the lungs where they cause fatal pulmonary emboli, a common cause of sudden chest pain and death. Warfarin can prevent these blood clots from forming.

Two genes determine how well a patient fares on warfarin. *CYP2C9* controls a liver enzyme responsible for breaking down warfarin, and *VKORC1* determines how sensitive you are to it. It turns out that warfarin complications arise from just eight variations in the *CYP2C9* gene and one in the *VKORC1* gene. In most cases a single nucleotide change determines whether warfarin works at all, works properly, or works too well.

In order to use the drug, doctors must administer a dose, monitor how quickly blood clots, and then painstakingly alter the dose until the blood clots quickly enough to prevent uncontrolled bleeding, but not so fast that clots form in the bloodstream. The body takes several days to respond to such changes.

Meanwhile, other drugs or even diet can affect warfarin level and activity. It's no wonder side effects of warfarin are responsible for one in ten hospital admissions in the U.S. costing the healthcare system over one billion dollars per year.

But now, prescribing warfarin may be guided by whether you have one of the mutations for these two genes, and the right dose more easily selected.

Prescribing small molecule drugs or biologics to more discreet populations is one obvious benefit of the advances made in unraveling the human genome. Designing new drugs based on trying to camouflage errors in the genome, genetic mutations, is another option that is now rapidly coming into play.

Nowhere will the ability to develop specifically targeted new drugs have more impact than for patients suffering from rare diseases. These estimated 14,000 distinct rare diseases differ greatly, but when taken together, a rare disease affects one in ten Americans, so it's likely that you know someone with a rare disease, whether you're aware of it or not. Approximately eighty percent of these rare diseases arise from defects in a single gene, and half of them affect children.

This single gene defect usually prevents the body from making a critical protein. When that protein serves as an enzyme, catalyzing vital biochemical reactions, replacing the enzyme becomes a valid treatment approach.

Several diseases can be treated this way. One example is Pompe's disease, which causes glycogen to accumulate in skeletal muscle and weakens the heart muscle. This ailment responds to the replacement of the enzyme, acid alpha-glucosidase.

Another ailment, Gaucher's disease, caused by the accumulation of certain fatty molecules, is treated with infusions of the glucocerebrosidase enzyme.

Enzyme replacement strategies work, but they aren't convenient. They must be administered regularly for the rest of your life. And many enzyme replacement therapies require intravenous infusions. In addition, in order to remain active, enzyme replacement therapies must be stored in carefully controlled environments.

Not only that. Enzyme replacement strategies can't address all single gene rare diseases because it may not be possible to get the drug to where it is needed inside the body.

For most diseases a better strategy would be to correct the protein defects when and where they are made.

But how do you do that?

The answer starts with RNA. The evolution of the RNA molecule is the reason we exist today. Life on earth, from the simplest bacterium to human beings, would have been impossible if RNA molecules hadn't been formed in the hot reactive stew of the primordial soup. They not only formed, but began to react with each other until they started replicating themselves. From RNA came DNA and protein. And with that, a sterile planet possessed the building blocks of life.

Throughout evolution, RNA has maintained its central role. Not merely as a go between, but an active, if mostly unseen, participant in any organism's life processes. That central role makes RNA the perfect location for some very targeted medicines.

Science first took notice of this complex but fragile molecule at the turn of the last century. By mid-20th century, the idea that RNA served as a messenger for protein production began to take hold. By the start of this century, science revealed critical roles for the molecule in biology, involving gene regulation, protein manufacture, and aging, among others.

The pace of research regarding this key molecule has accelerated since Andrew Fire and Craig Mellow received the Nobel Prize for Medicine in 2006, for work reported in 1998, that genes could be silenced by interfering with their RNA.

At the turn of this century, according to Muhammad Sohail, editor of the Journal of RNAi and Gene Silencing, there were only 70 to 80 papers in this esoteric field, but midway through the last decade, the number had leapt to 70 to 80 every hour! Over the same period the number of biotech companies looking to exploit this evolving science has also rocketed.

Because RNA is the link between the cell's instructions housed in the nucleus and its activity beyond in the cytoplasm, interfering with or altering RNA's function can have sweeping impacts on how the cell interprets the instructions from its own DNA.

Knowing how to interfere with RNA opens the door for us to prevent disease before it can begin.

There are a number of different strategies for doing this. They all rely on the RNA molecule's similarity to DNA.

DNA exists as two long separate but intertwined strands held together by weak bonds of attraction between complementary bases, adenine (A), cytosine (C), guanine (G), and thymine (T). The genetic code arises because A always pairs with T and C always pairs with G.

RNA, on the other hand, is a single-strand molecule comprised of the bases adenine (A), cytosine (C), guanine (G), all of which are part of DNA, and uracil (U), a base that is very similar to thymine. While RNA is a single strand, it loops around and folds back on itself in such a way that A always pairs with U and C always pairs with G. As noted in the last chapter, the fact that both molecules are comprised of complementary bases means that the mobile RNA can ferry out (from the cell's nucleus) the genetic information contained in the stationary DNA.

The ability of RNA and DNA to bind to each other can be exploited to interrupt cellular processes by employing very small snippets of DNA called oligomers or oligonucleotides. Whereas a single human gene is, on average, comprised of at least three thousand nucleotide units, an oligomer is usually comprised of ten to thirty units.

When an oligomer binds to RNA, it can interrupt cellular activity. That proves useful when a cell's activity has gone awry.

In 1978, Paul Zamecnik and Mary Stephenson, both of Harvard University Medical School, created the first active oligomer aimed at a virus that causes cancer in chickens.

That virus was first discovered by Peyton Rous of the Rockefeller University in 1911. Rous took a tumor from a chicken, ground it up with salt water and filtered it through such a fine filter that no cells, either chicken or bacteria, remained. Rous then injected the "cell-free" extract into chickens. The injected chickens developed a type of cancer, a sarcoma to be exact. He dubbed whatever agent was causing chicken cells to transform into cancer cells the Rous Sarcoma Virus. It was the very first virus discovered that causes cancer. Rous received the Nobel Prize in Physiology or Medicine over fifty years later, in 1966, as a result of this discovery.

In the time between the discovery of the Rous Sarcoma Virus and Zamecnik and Stephenson's experiments, it had been established that viruses are comprised of some structural proteins and genetic material, either DNA or RNA, and that they rely on the cellular machinery of the host cell, the ribosome, to produce proteins. The Rous Sarcoma Virus in particular is an RNA virus.

Zamecnik and Stephenson prevented the Rous Sarcoma Virus from transforming chicken cells into cancer cells. They used a 13-base oligonucleotide that bound to the RNA of the virus. This was the first time a small DNA molecule, complementary to a section of RNA, was used to interrupt cellular processes. The oligonucleotide bound to the viral RNA preventing it from engaging the chicken's ribosome. This stopped the chicken cells from producing the proteins needed to cause the cancer to form and grow.

The experiment by these Harvard scientists marked the birth of "antisense therapy" and made it possible to make targeted medicines (Figure 2.1, #11).

As mentioned in the previous chapter, copying instructions from DNA isn't an entirely straightforward activity, at least for creatures more complex than bacteria. When the cell needs instructions from DNA, an enzyme in the nucleus known as RNA polymerase (Figure 3.3) begins to copy the instructions by peeling open the strands of DNA and manufacturing a strand of RNA, base by base, that is the perfect complement to the unzipped DNA strand; every A on the DNA is incorporated as a U in RNA, every C in the DNA is represented by G in the RNA, every T in the DNA becomes an A in the RNA and every G in the DNA shows up as a C in the growing RNA strand.

The problem is that, like in any good book, first drafts need a bit of editing. Genes don't reside on the chromosome in one contiguous piece. Interspersed throughout are sections of DNA that don't code for protein. In most cases we don't know yet what these sections do.

In order to make a protein, the cell must edit out all of these non-essential sections, called introns, from the growing strand of RNA and splice together only the protein coding portions, called exons. The RNA cannot move out of the nucleus as a mature message for the protein coding machinery, the ribosome, until all of the introns are removed.

While it still has introns, the RNA is a pre-messenger molecule, and is confined to within the nucleus.

For a surprising number of diseases, especially rare diseases, a single defect in just one of those exons is enough to cause the protein manufactured to fail to work properly. Sometimes, the defect will cause the ribosome to stop dead in its tracks and fail to make the protein altogether.

According to the World Health Organization, ten babies in every one thousand have a single gene disease, with over four thousand diseases caused by a single defective gene. A Canadian paper (Scriver, 1995) reported that so called monogenic disease may be responsible for up to 40% of children being seen in hospitals.

Some cases of cystic fibrosis and Duchenne muscular dystrophy are caused by these "nonsense" mutations that stop the production of protein. The mutation can be a single nucleotide change in just one of the DNA's exons.

We also know that in seventy percent of neurological disorders, the process of splicing the exons together has failed or is altered.

Other times, the instructions dictate that the cellular machinery incorporates the wrong amino acid into the growing protein and the protein folds improperly. It becomes useless or imperfect, affecting other cellular processes.

For example, take sickle cell anemia. A change of a single base of DNA causes the wrong amino acid to be inserted into the hemoglobin protein. In this case, valine is inserted instead of glutamic acid. Valine and glutamic acid couldn't be more different. Glutamic acid, the correct amino acid, is water loving, while valine, the wrong one, abhors water.

When valine is inserted into hemoglobin protein, the surrounding water in our bodies repels it and distorts the shape of the protein. As a result, the red blood cell becomes elongated, sickle-shaped and stiff, rather than the normal flexible, round, and smooth doughnut shape. That sickle-shaped cell gets stuck in small blood vessels. In addition, sickle cells fail to carry oxygen efficiently, causing painful crises for those who suffer from the disease.

Since the early 1970s when Theodore Friedman and Richard Roblin first suggested that defective DNA could be replaced with "good" DNA, scientists have been working on "gene therapies" to do just that.

Many scientists have focused on replacing genes wholesale by inserting a new, correct copy of the gene into cells using viruses as the carrier. It's a thought-provoking approach. However, researchers have run up against several obstacles. Getting the gene into the cells that need it, avoiding the body's immune defenses, and finding a way to make the gene function properly have all been huge challenges.

Other work has focused on inserting stem cells into host tissue where they can mature into healthy versions of the adult cells and replace the diseased cells.

At the same time, building on Zamecnik's work with Rous sarcoma virus, other scientists have started attacking the problem of faulty

DNA, not by fixing the DNA, but by blocking the message coming from that DNA from being transmitted. In other words, camouflaging or patching the message.

As of this writing, we don't know how to go into a cell and correct a small defect in a strand of messenger RNA. That doesn't mean we can't camouflage the message using the same "antisense" therapy that Zamecnik employed. In the same way you use makeup to be more attractive, the message from the gene in the nucleus can be camouflaged to be more "attractive" to the ribosome in the outer part of the cell.

The first way to stymie damaging RNA, either from disease causing genes or from acquired viruses, is by destroying their message. Zamecnik showed that when an oligomer was attached to Rous sarcoma virus RNA, the virus failed to replicate itself and couldn't cause cancer.

Here's why that effort was successful. When the DNA oligomer binds to the viral RNA, the ribosome can't manufacture proteins. The enzymes, which are constantly seeking to tidy up stray bits of bound nucleic acids, destroy both the RNA and the oligomer binding to it. The protein manufacturing system is free and able to respond to other messenger RNA strands. The message is blocked.

Scientists use this technique either to stop a defective protein from being made or to damp down the excessive manufacture of a protein that is harmful to the body.

While destroying bad messages will suppress the production of disease causing proteins, the same process won't help if you want to start the supply of a missing, functional protein. To generate the protein, the ribosome *needs* to get the instructions.

The second way to prevent RNA causing disease is to change, or camouflage, the message it conveys. By aiming small bits of antisense DNA at pre-messenger RNA, we can create slight changes to the mature messenger RNA that leaves the nucleus, thus altering what happens in a cell. The RNA is not destroyed, and neither is the oligomer, because the enzyme clean up team does not recognize it and fails to tidy it up. The message gets through to the ribosome but it has been altered, beneficially.

Scattered throughout the genes that encode for proteins are sections of information unnecessary for producing those proteins, the introns. These oligomers take advantage of that fact. When mature messenger RNA is transcribed from the DNA template, it must first knit together the protein coding exons and cut out the non–coding introns. This process is called splicing. After splicing, the messenger RNA can move from the nucleus to the protein producing ribosomes in the outer part of the cell.

A collection of proteins and small nuclear RNAs accomplish this task by identifying where each exon and intron starts and stops on the strand of pre-messenger RNA. They must cut the pre-messenger RNA at the precise boundary between each exon and intron. Finally, they splice together the exons in the correct order. Though this process may sound complicated, the cells in our bodies splice messenger RNA millions and millions of times a day.

While they have the ability to splice out introns and the information they contain, the cells can't excise defects found within exons. Any problems in the coding sections for proteins remain once the mature messenger RNA has been spliced together. If the problem within the exon leads to a minor change from one amino acid to another that shares similar chemical properties, the result could be imperceptible. For example, a water-loving amino acid could be swapped for another water-loving amino acid by the ribosome.

If the amino acids exchanged are more dissimilar, as in the defect associated with sickle cell anemia, the protein may not function correctly and could cause disease. If the defect in a particular exon causes the ribosome to stop making protein altogether, it will almost certainly cause disease.

However, what if a protein doesn't actually need all of the amino acids in the complete protein for it to be active and viable? What if entire exons could be hidden from the splicing process? In the earlier analogy about a car, it might still work and be drivable but have a coat of paint missing or a different radio.

A shorter strand of messenger RNA would result, without the defective exon, and an active, or even partially active protein could still result. In that case, finding a way to skip over an exon with a defect may allow a new, functioning protein, albeit slightly shorter than the natural protein, to be produced. This would be especially true of a defect that orders the ribosome to stop during the processing phase.

It turns out that the cells in our bodies "skip" exons all the time. That truth flies in the face of genetic dogma established in the 1930s and 1940s, when it was thought that one gene produces one protein, often an enzyme. However, for possibly 95% of multi-exon genes, the cell can splice messenger RNA together in several remarkably different ways.

Take, for example, the hormone calcitonin, which is produced by the thyroid gland and is critical for the regulation of calcium in the bloodstream. The calcitonin gene contains 6 exons. However, in order to produce calcitonin, thyroid cells splice down the pre-messenger RNA so that the mature message includes only exons 1, 2, 3 and 4 (Figure 4.1)

That doesn't mean exons 5 and 6 serve no purpose. Different cells in the nervous system take the same pre-messenger RNA produced from the calcitonin gene and skip exon 4. By splicing exons 1, 2, 3, 5 and 6 together to make a different mRNA, the ribosomes for the nervous system generate a different protein product, alpha-calcitonin gene-related peptide, or a-CGRP, that relaxes blood vessels.

Another example of normal alternative splicing occurs in the AMPA receptor that was described first by Danish medicinal chemist and neurobiologist, Tage Honore, in 1982. AMPA stands for alpha-amino-3-hydroxy-5-methyl-4-isoxazolepropionic acid. It is a very important receptor in the brain, composed of four subunits which each have two forms – a "flip" form which makes the AMPA receptors have high activity, and a "flop" form which makes low activity receptors. The flip and flop forms are mutually exclusive and are formed by an alternatively spliced section of the pre-mRNA - either splicing out exon 3 but leaving exon 4 in the mature mRNA or splicing in exon 3 but leaving out exon 4. The high activity AMPA receptor leads to excessive excitability of the central nervous system, causing diseases like epilepsy or amyotrophic lateral sclerosis or ALS (Lou Gehrig's disease).

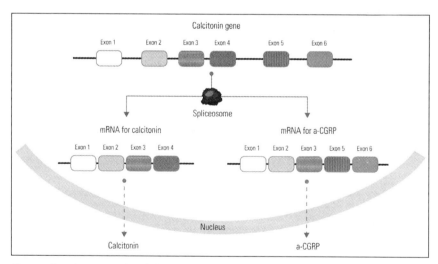

Figure 4.1. An example of alternative splicing. The calcitonin gene is composed of six exons. In the nucleus of thyroid gland cells, exons 1, 2, 3, and 4 are spliced together, the mRNA leaves the nucleus and the ribosome generates calcitonin from these instructions. The same pre-mRNA strand in the nucleus of nervous system cells has a different fate. Exons 1, 2, 3, 5, and 6 are spliced together to form a different mRNA strand that leaves the nucleus, is then read by the ribosome and leads to the generation of alpha-calcitonin gene-related peptide.

Several other nasty neuromuscular diseases are linked to mRNA splicing defects, so the opportunity to effectively, safely, and consistently alter splicing beneficially has wide ranging implications.

Sometimes, skipping an exon doesn't necessarily change the job a protein does. Instead, it affects how well the job gets done.

Alternative splicing is not just confined to humans. All animals and plants utilize alternative splicing to make multiple proteins from any single gene. Much of the scientific work on alternative splicing has been done in *Arabidopsis*, a small, annual, spring flowering plant from Europe, Asia and northwest Africa. Because *Arabidopsis* has a relatively short life cycle of six weeks, and a small genome of only 157 million base pairs, botanists and geneticists routinely use it to study alternative splicing.

The fruit fly has also been an important research subject. An extreme example of alternative splicing was described in 2004 where it was found that a single gene of the fruit fly, *Dscam,* gives rise to 38,016 different mRNA variants and proteins.

Because alternative splicing is well documented in nature, it makes sense that modern medicine would attempt to trigger that mechanism to produce effective proteins.

By using oligomers, we can alter the way a pre-messenger RNA splices together its exons. RNA splicing takes place when a collection of RNA/protein complexes recognizes a specific sequence of bases, the four letters A, C, G and U, at the interface between introns and exons as well as sequences within the intron. These complexes, called spliceosomes, cause the RNA to loop around, putting the exons in close proximity to each other. Then, they cut the intron out and stitch, or splice, the adjoining exons together.

If the pre-messenger RNA doesn't contain the specific bases signaling the junction between an intron and an exon, the spliceosome can't recognize it and can't splice together the correct exons. That's where therapeutic oligomers come in. Suppose you have a gene with six exons and five introns, of which exon 4 contains a nonsense mutation that you want to skip in order to make a functioning protein. By creating an oligomer that is complementary to the splice site at the beginning of exon 4, you can effectively camouflage or mask that splice site from being recognized by the busy spliceosome.

When the spliceosome begins processing the pre-messenger RNA, the oligomer will hide exon 4.

Instead of splicing exon 3 and exon 4 together, the spliceosome will create a messenger RNA comprised of exon 3 spliced to exon 5, skipping exon 4 altogether. The protein will then be shorter, missing the amino acids that would have been coded for by a non-mutated exon 4, but potentially retaining important activity.

In fact, it is possible to produce an effective protein with missing sections. Doing so offers the opportunity to address some of the most vexing genetic conditions that afflict humans today.

But how did we get to the point where we can literally defy our DNA?

In the century and a half since an Augustinian friar nudged open the door to the age of genetics by publishing his efforts to breed sweet peas, medicine has changed dramatically. At the same time that Gregor Johann Mendel (1822-1884) was untangling the basic tenets of genetic inheritance, Louis Pasteur (1822-1895) was first proposing the idea that infections, the principal killer at the time, were caused not by an imbalance of humors, but the spread of germs. That theory spawned medical advances that include sanitation, aseptic surgical techniques, and antibiotics, as well as the pasteurization of milk that pays tribute to the great Frenchman. It is not an overstatement to say that these advances have resulted in decades being added to the life expectancies of people living in developed countries.

Mendel's work on genes, however, is only now beginning to provoke such a revolution. His efforts moldered for roughly thirty years before they were rediscovered and applied to understanding human inheritance and genetic conditions. It took another forty years before scientists were certain that DNA was the source of genes and inheritance in humans. Not until Watson and Crick announced the structure of DNA in 1953 did the pace of genetic discoveries begin to accelerate. Researchers went from describing the central dogma that DNA stores genetic information and RNA provides the template from which proteins are made, to deciphering the genetic code and identifying the specific genetic defects associated with disease.

Though the field of genomics started 150 years ago, it has not yet been fully integrated into drug development. Until now, that has proven prohibitively expensive and time consuming.

But that's changing.

This change is important because the field of drug development is rife with stories of drugs that show remarkable promise in early studies, until serious, but rare side effects show up when the drug is tested in larger groups of patients. Historically in these situations, pharmaceutical companies often halt development or pull the drug off the market.

But everyone involved with the creation of the drug wonders what made it work so well for some yet prove dangerous for others.

Let's take a look at the story of Vioxx.

Vioxx is a non-steroidal anti-inflammatory drug (NSAID) that was often prescribed for arthritis. It's like aspirin and ibuprofen, as well as more than thirty other effective drugs that share the common and serious side effect of stomach ulcers.

But unlike the others, Vioxx doesn't cause ulcers. Here's why.

The body uses inflammation as the first line of defense in fighting infection. A critical step in the inflammation process is the production of the chemicals prostaglandin and thromboxane, employing two different pathways, cyclooxygenase-1 (COX-1) and cyclooxygenase-2 (COX-2). Most cells in our bodies employ the COX-1 pathway that is essential for the cells to be healthy. The COX-2 pathway turns on only in specific cells in areas of inflammation, especially when joints are inflamed.

NSAIDs work by blocking both COX pathways. Stifling the COX-2 pathway effectively reduces joint inflammation. But the stomach relies on prostaglandin to protect it from stomach acid and inhibiting the COX-1 pathway reduces the level of protective prostaglandin in the stomach lining, leading to irritation, ulcers, and in severe cases bleeding or perforation.

The scientists who created Vioxx hoped that blocking only the COX-2 pathway might reduce the inflammatory prostaglandins and thromboxane while protecting the stomach by leaving the COX-1 pathway unaffected.

In 1998, Merck submitted a new drug application documenting all of the laboratory, animal and human testing data pertaining to the development of Vioxx. In 1999, the FDA approved Vioxx for sale in the U.S., with the caveat common to most drugs: that the company formally study it over a longer period of time in more patients in addition to the standard requirement to monitor sales, collect data on side effects, and report back.

Post approval studies are designed to test drugs in "real life" settings thereby helping to define the true incidence of rare side effects. Merck conducted several such studies. In 2000, the *New England Journal of Medicine* published the results of the Vioxx gastrointestinal outcome research study. It suggested a small, but significant, increase in the risk of heart attack over twelve months. While only one out of every thousand taking the traditional NSAID, naproxen, had a heart attack, with Vioxx, four out of every thousand suffered that fate.

Despite warnings about this increased risk, by 2003, Vioxx reached blockbuster status, with annual sales of $2.5 billion.

The following September, Merck concluded that the risk of a heart attack was simply too high and voluntarily removed Vioxx from the market. The results of other studies haven't conclusively answered whether the risks for heart disease outweigh the benefits of reduced stomach ulcers. In 2005, regulatory panels in the U.S. and Canada urged Merck to bring Vioxx back with a specific warning about heart attacks. Merck declined.

When scientists developed the COX-2 inhibitors they didn't appreciate that by blocking the COX-2 pathway alone, they might be altering the balance between prostaglandins and thromboxane throughout the body, including in the heart and blood vessels supplying the heart.

Yet, the question remains: Why did the Vioxx work well for so many patients but cause grievous harm, in this case a heart attack, to a select group?

So far, nobody knows. I believe it is likely that a gene controls this outcome. Once identified, the availability of personal genome sequencing will permit physicians to predict if any of the COX-2 inhibitors are likely to cause a heart attack and prescribe just to those not at risk.

When such a gene is discovered, it will probably be too late for Vioxx.

Many blockbuster drugs cause rare or common side effects as a result of personal genetic differences. Four drugs, the antidepressant fluoxetine (Prozac), the anti-acid reflux drug Propulsid, the diabetes drug Avandia and macrolide antibiotics similar to erythromycin, can alter the electrical changes in your heart, prolong the QT interval and in rare circumstances cause heart attacks.

Scanning the genome for genetic predisposition to side effects can and will become standard practice during drug development and in routine clinical care as medicine advances and becomes more personalized.

QT Interval Prolongation

If you have a mutation in a gene that regulates the electrical activity of your heart, taking Propulsid or erythromycin can provoke a heart attack. The genes that put you at risk, *KCNQ1/KCNE1* (LQT1) and *NaV1.5* (LQT3), follow the rules of dominant inheritance. You only need to inherit one gene from one of your parents in order to be at risk of a heart attack from taking erythromycin.

The electrical record of a heart contraction, the electrocardiogram, has several distinct peaks and troughs on it, called the P wave (the electrical wave spreading across the upper chambers or atria), the QRS complex (the electrical wave passing through the muscle of the ventricles causing them to contract and pump the blood out and into the lungs and around the body) and the T wave (the heart muscle re-polarizing in preparation for the next beat). The shapes, amplitudes and durations of these various electrical waves, and the interval between them, are well defined. Changes to any one of these parameters can indicate disease.

Propulsid, after it became generally available, was recognized as a drug that could, for some people, lengthen the interval between the Q and T waves, sometimes causing fatal changes in electrical activity in the heart. As a result of that increased knowledge, all new drugs now have to undergo testing to see if they cause QT prolongation. Propulsid was withdrawn from the U.S. market in 2000 because there are alternative drugs that can be used to treat acid reflux. Still, screening for these genetic conditions becomes important if you have an infection that could respond to erythromycin. Then, your doctor could use the tools of genomics to predict if you are at risk of side effects before deciding whether or not to prescribe it.

Some of those abandoned drugs could be resurrected if a genetic cause for their side effects could be identified. That would provide a test to ensure the drug is safe for an individual patient. This is expensive, time consuming, and not readily available until now. In the future, more companies will attempt this if the drug in question promises to meet a hitherto unmet medical need.

With the cost of genomic sequencing rapidly declining, genetic information will become a critical component of clinical trials for all potential new drugs, not just those with an already identified rare adverse effects. As some patients respond positively to a particular agent and others develop side effects, the researchers conducting the trial will search for genetic differences as a possible explanation. If genetics is indeed the cause, when a company submits the data for a new drug for approval, they will document who is genetically most likely to suffer. When the drug comes to market, physicians will be able to tailor their prescriptions to the genetic makeup of the individual patient.

At that time, the era of the blockbuster drugs will be over. Precisely identifying genetic profiles means that pharmaceutical companies will develop new drugs for smaller groups of patients. They will specifically target the genetic source of disease and develop drugs that can stop a disease literally at birth. New drugs will treat fewer patients, but each patient will be treated for longer and from a younger age, with greater safety, to prevent the disease in the first place.

We are truly on the path to a "predict and prevent paradigm" of personalized medicine.

Some day in the future, everyone who is born will be given both a birth certificate and a genetic map. At that time, we will be able to address some of the most vexing inherited conditions that afflict humans today.

In so doing, we will indeed be able to defy our DNA

Summary

Over the 35 years since Zamecnik experimented with the first oligonucleotide to block viral RNA, we have come a long way. Alternative splicing is now understood to be the body's way of translating 25,000 genes into 150,000 proteins.

A single altered gene, exon or even nucleotide can have fundamental and lethal effects. Modern medicine is now developing the necessary tools to effectively start turning the tide on these faulty genes. Therapeutic oligomers will allow us to effectively treat diseases, even before their message leaves the nucleus on its way to the cellular factory.

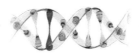

Chapter Five

The End of
Hereditary Rare Disease

When I was a family doctor back in England in the 80s and 90s, I had at least one patient with a rare disease on my list of three thousand patients. Anthony Michaels lived with his devoted mother in a small, modern, two-bedroom house on the other side of town. Anthony had cystic fibrosis. In those days he had a life expectancy of only sixteen years.

Anthony was in and out of the big regional hospital in Birmingham (England's second biggest city) every few weeks, and indeed he had a schedule of admissions prearranged so that he could receive intense courses of intravenous antibiotics and physical therapy to help clear the sticky plugs of mucus blocking his airways that is characteristic of cystic fibrosis.

Despite these regular admissions, Anthony would frequently succumb to some new chest infection, his breathing would deteriorate, his cough would get worse, and his temperature would climb. He would be rushed into the hospital for emergency courses of his usual treatment of powerful intravenous antibiotics and to be put on a breathing machine.

When I would see him a few weeks later, he would look emaciated but both he and his mum would be joking and playfully teasing me, despite the knowledge that as a teenager, he was now only expected to live another year or two.

One day, I was asked by the specialist pediatric pulmonologist at the big regional center, who looked after about thirty children with CF, whether I would give Anthony "home intravenous antibiotic therapy." What that meant was that I (or one of the competent and experienced district nurses) would have to go into the Michaels' home, put an intravenous line with a powerful antibiotic (gentamicin, if my memory is correct) into one of Anthony's fragile veins, and after a period of observation to ensure all was well, remove the IV access and tidy up.

In those days, there were no inhaled antibiotics and although Anthony daily took many capsules of the vital pancreatic enzyme supplements that he required, there was no effective treatment to keep the lungs clear of the nasty bacteria, especially *Pseudomonas aeruginosa*, which he therefore harbored in low levels even on the best of days. On bad days, the number of these nasty bugs would surge and down he would go with the next chest infection. Inevitably, a day would come when the bacteria would become resistant to the lifesaving, high doses of gentamicin he received.

I agreed to provide "domiciliary IV antibiotic care" for Anthony, although it had not been "approved" or become standard practice at that time. Already the expensive drugs I prescribed to keep Anthony alive had attracted some concern from the local healthcare administrators and few other GPs within the West Midlands region, covering a large part of central England, had agreed to give IV antibiotics to their CF patients at home, preferring them to journey in to the regional center for their regular weekly course.

Over the years, Anthony had a series of setbacks, and he had several operations for squints, unrelated to his breathing and digestive problems. I left my practice, but my guess is that he would surely have been one of those to receive the life enhancing cycling inhaled tobramycin antibiotic (TOBI, a cousin of gentamicin) by nebulizer, which contributed to life expectancy doubling to 32 years. He would probably have been eventually listed for a lung or double lung or even a heart-lung transplant.

For several years, I worked as a drug development physician at Chiron Corporation (acquired by Novartis in 2005), which was working with TOBI for CF and another pulmonary disease, bronchiectasis. Chiron then moved on to work on a project using a drug to prevent lung transplant rejection. The memory of Anthony's cheeky grin and bubbly sense of humor always reminded me of what physicians in the pharmaceutical industry are trying to achieve: the development of drugs that will add years of good quality life to people like Anthony.

I believe that Anthony did indeed receive a heart-lung transplant, but that he did not long survive that procedure.

Anthony was one of the patients whose humor and fortitude in the face of adversity, and with little hope of living a normal life span or quality of life, inspired me as a doctor. At least a firm diagnosis had been made and although there was then no definitive treatment, his mother and he were told what to expect.

I had other patients who had no diagnosis at all. They had strange conditions and were repeatedly examined by top specialists who agreed something was amiss, but couldn't tell what it was. In this new era of genomics, many of these rare diseases, alas most still lacking any effective treatment, can at least be accurately diagnosed and the specific genetic mutation identified. And many more of these rare diseases will soon no doubt be revealed.

Currently about seven thousand rare diseases have been character-ized and the faulty gene isolated. There are estimated to be at least another seven thousand which have not yet had a causative genetic mutation identified, and thus are untreatable, but gradually these diseases will be understood.

Most of these rare genetic disorders are only diagnosed once the patient has developed symptoms of the disorder, bringing him or her to the attention of doctors. And because these diseases are due to faulty genes, the child is destined to develop the disease from the moment they are conceived, literally, when the father's sperm meets the mother's egg.

These genetic diseases are unlikely ever to be fully preventable, although many can be screened for in early pregnancy, with the option for the parents to end the pregnancy of an affected embryo. The next step for those babies is to develop effective treatments for these rare and often lethal diseases.

I believe that oligomers may be a potential answer for many of these.

I, too, am a parent affected by a rare disease. Multicystic dysplastic kidney (MCDK) is a rare disease occurring in one in roughly 4,300 births. Babies born with one dysplastic kidney can survive well on the remaining normal kidney. Ten weeks before he was born, one of my own sons was detected with this rare defect. Unfortunately, he appeared to have a blockage affecting his other kidney, meaning neither of his kidneys would work. Within hours of his birth he was subject to an operation to try and bypass his blocked kidney, but alas the operation failed. He was brought from the operating theater to me and I was given the news that he was expected to die within the next twenty-four hours. I was left to cuddle this little bundle in a hospital cubicle, miles away from where his mother was recovering from giving birth to him. Against the odds, he survived the day, the night and then the next day. After several operations to re-plumb his solitary, working, but now damaged kidney and then remove his non-functioning one, he survived childhood with blood pressure treatment, treatment for the side effects of that treatment and various supplements. So, yes, I know from personal experience how rare disease can affect a family.

There is no single, widely accepted definition for rare diseases. Some definitions rely solely on the number of people living with a disease. Other definitions include other factors, such as the lack of adequate treatment; the severity of the disease; or a lack of resources to care for the patient. Some people prefer the term orphan disease and use it as a synonym for rare disease, such as the European Organization for Rare Diseases (EURORDIS) which combines both rare diseases and neglected diseases (those with no treatment available) into a larger category of "orphan diseases."

The orphan drug movement began in the U.S. over thirty years ago. It was the moving force behind the Orphan Drug Act (ODA) of 1983, a federal law designed to encourage research into rare diseases and possible cures. The ODA includes both rare diseases and any non-rare diseases "for which there is no reasonable expectation that the cost of developing and making a drug available in the U.S. for such disease or condition will [be] recovered from its sales in the U.S." as orphan diseases. Since 1983, more than 2,200 drugs have entered the research pipeline and more than 360 have completed their development and been approved for marketing. Currently orphan products account for about one third of all New Molecular Entities being approved.

The subsequent Rare Disease Act of 2002 defines rare disease strictly according to prevalence, specifically "any disease or condition that affects less than 200,000 persons in the United States," or about one in 1,500 people. Prevalence is defined as the total number of cases of the disease in the population at a given time, or the total number of cases in the population divided by the number of individuals in the population. It is used as an estimate of how common a disease is within a population at a certain point in time. This should not be confused with incidence (the number of new diagnoses in a given year), which is used to describe the impact of rare diseases.

The increased regulatory attention afforded to rare diseases led to the U.S. Food and Drug Administration (FDA)'s Center for Drug Evaluation and Research (CDER) establishing a Rare Disease Program in February 2010, with its own Associate Director of Rare Diseases (ADRD) reporting to the Director of the Office of New Drugs (OND). This new team was given the goal of facilitating and supporting the research, development, regulation and approval of drugs for the treatment of rare disorders, and was to complement the work of FDA's Office of Orphan Product Development (OOPD). It would become the focal point of contact at FDA for Rare Disease stakeholders, such as companies developing small molecule drugs, oligomers and biologics and patient advocacy organizations. The rare disease program team would facilitate interactions with CDER and their sister Center of Biologic Evaluation and Research (CBER). The ADRD would help drug development companies navigate complex regulatory requirements and the increasingly intricate bureaucracy that is the FDA. There is still much to do. Currently, only about two hundred of the seven thousand characterized rare diseases in the U.S. have an approved treatment available.

I have worked on several rare disease programs during my twenty years as a physician in the pharmaceutical industry, and led numerous interactions with regulators in the U.S. (FDA) and Europe (European Medicines Agency or EMA). I am pleased that in some cases the new drug applications that I worked on have already been submitted and approved. I suspect that the increased FDA focus on rare diseases will indeed lead to faster development programs and more approval for ground-breaking pharmaceutical products, and hopefully oligomers, in the years ahead.

The key to understanding FDA structure, roles and responsibility as it pertains to rare disease is to understand the complementary but distinct separation between the Office of Orphan Medicinal Products (OOPD) and the Office of New Drugs (OND)'s Rare Disease Program (RDP), which can be summarized this way (Figure 5.1):

OOPD	OND RDP
➢ Administrates the ODA • Designations • Exclusivity • Orphan grants	➢ Facilitates communication within CDER/OND review divisions
➢ Device programs	➢ Focuses on complex regulatory requirements for INDs*, NDAs* and BLAs*
➢ Pediatric focus	➢ Develops policy, procedures and advice for rare disease clinical development programs
➢ Strong advocacy work with rare disease stakeholders	
Common areas: coordinate communication across FDA centers and offices, and with outside stakeholders; enhance rare disease information available on FDA website	

* ODA =Orphan Drug Act. IND =Investigational New Drug (the application to the FDA to allow initial human testing). NDA = New Drug Application (the enormous dossier containing all the research, animal testing, clinical studies, manufacturing and quality testing that the FDA reviews prior to approving the product suitable for marketing). BLA = Biologic License Application (the NDA for biologic products).

Figure 5.1. The similarities and differences between the FDA's Office of Orphan Medicinal Products (OOPD) and the Office of New Drug's Rare Disease Program (OND RDP)

Further evidence of the increasing FDA interest in rare diseases is provided by the seven rare disease approvals (three drugs and four biologics) in the first nine months of 2010 (Appendix B) of a total of 17 New Molecular Entities (NMEs) approved (ten drugs as NDAs and seven biologics as BLAs).

In Japan, the legal definition of a rare disease is one that affects fewer than 50,000 patients in Japan, or about one in 2,500 people. The European definition of a rare disease is a life-threatening or chronically debilitating disease that is of such low prevalence that special combined efforts are needed to address it. The term "low prevalence" is later defined as generally meaning fewer than one in 2,000 people, consistent with the European Commission's definition of rare. Diseases that are statistically rare, but not also life-threatening, chronically debilitating, or inadequately treated, are excluded from their definition. The definitions used in the medical literature and by national health plans are similarly divided, with definitions ranging from one in a thousand to one in two hundred thousand. The Global Genes Project estimates there are some 350 million people worldwide currently affected with a rare disease.

Although each individual rare disease is rare by definition, the sheer number of different, individual rare diseases results in approximately eight percent of the population of the European Union being affected by a rare disease, close to the estimated ten percent of U.S. patients who are similarly suspected of suffering from a rare disorder. Most rare diseases are genetic, and thus are present throughout the person's entire life, even if symptoms do not immediately appear. However, many rare diseases appear early in life, and about thirty percent of children with rare diseases will die before reaching their fifth birthday. Rare diseases can vary in prevalence between populations, so a disease that is rare in some populations may be common in others. This is especially true of genetic diseases and infectious diseases. An example is cystic fibrosis (CF), a genetic disease, which is relatively common in Caucasian Europeans. The recessive gene is carried by approximately one in 25 people. For the disease to occur both copies of the gene must be affected. Thus 1/25 x 1/25 partnerships are likely to result in two carriers coming together (i.e. one in 625 partnerships). These parents have a one in four chance that their child will receive the recessive gene from both partners. This gives an incidence of one in 4 x 625 new births = one in 2,500. In Asians, CF is even rarer.

Finland has a higher prevalence of about forty rare diseases; these are known collectively as the Finnish disease heritage. Ashkenazi Jews also have a higher prevalence of certain rare diseases with an estimated one in four individuals being a carrier of one of several genetic conditions, including Tay-Sachs Disease, Canavan, Niemann-Pick, Gaucher, Familial Dysautonomia, Bloom Syndrome, Fanconi anemia and Mucolipidosis IV.

There are many companies whose development programs now focus on rare or orphan diseases including Synageva BioPharma Corp. (based in Massachusetts), Swedish Orphan Biovitrum, Shire plc (British), Genzyme (also based in Massachusetts but recently acquired by the French giant, Sanofi Aventis), Lundbeck (a Danish company) and BioMarin (a small California based company). Disappointing as it is that there has not been more work conducted on rare diseases in the past, it is encouraging to learn how much research is now underway. Perhaps discoveries in rare diseases will have much greater impact to future healthcare than is expected.

Take the example of progeria. Progeria is a very rare disease affecting about one in four million people. It is now known to be caused by a single base change from a C to a T in the middle of the Lamin A gene

(*LMNA*). This causes 150 nucleotides in exon eleven to be spliced out of the final mRNA, and the resulting abnormal protein lacks fifty amino acids. The disease, also known by its longer title of Hutchinson-Gilford progeria syndrome (HGPS), results in rapid aging (at about seven times the normal rate) and children dying usually around age 12 to13 years from a heart attack, by which time they look like they are in their eighties.

The molecular biology behind progeria was characterized some years ago, with a buildup of a toxic protein (progerin) in the cells that led to the premature heart disease. In an experimental mouse model, the toxic protein could be reduced by treatment with a farnesyl transferase inhibitor (FTI) drug (lonafarnib), and the mice survived without the premature cardiovascular disease.

Since 2007, a clinical trial has been underway in progeria to see if the same drug will also work in the human disease, although the ClinicalTrial.Gov website for this study (run by Schering-Plough and the Progeria Research Foundation at Boston Children's hospital) has not been updated since December 2007. At that time, the study was slated to complete in October 2009. There are only 42 identified children in the world (from at least 15 countries – including Pakistan, Croatia, Korea, Argentina and Venezuela) with this rare condition making the conduct of this clinical study incredibly challenging. Having been in touch with the Progeria Research Foundation in mid 2012, I understand that the results from this study will be publically released soon. I hope they are positive.

In addition, it has been found that the toxic protein does build up in the cells of the elderly, so perhaps a better understanding of the rare disease progeria will have future important implications for aging in general. Maybe in time, it will be possible to skip the point mutation in the precursor mRNA with an oligomer and create a different mRNA that will be much closer to the normal message, with most of the 150 missing nucleotides restored. This could conceivably prevent the buildup of the abnormal progerin and the devastating disease progeria.

William Harvey was best known for determining how the circulatory system worked, but in 1657 he remarked in a letter about rare diseases: "Nature is nowhere accustomed more openly to display her secret mysteries than in cases where she shows tracings of her workings beside the beaten path; nor is there any better way to advance the proper practice of medicine that to give our minds to the discovery of the usual law of Nature by careful investigation of cases of rare forms of diseases. For it has been found in almost all things, that what they contain of useful or applicable nature is hardly perceived unless we are deprived of them, or they become deranged in some way."

Many infectious diseases are prevalent in a given geographic area but rare everywhere else, usually limited by the distribution of specific climatic conditions or certain animals required for their life cycle, or both. Other diseases, such as many rare forms of cancer, have no apparent pattern of distribution but are simply rare. The classification of other conditions depends in part on the population being studied: All forms of cancer in children are generally considered rare, because so few children develop cancer, but the same cancer in adults may be more common. With a single diagnosed patient only, ribose-5-phosphate isomerase deficiency is presently considered the rarest genetic disease. The distribution of disease areas that were targeted for an orphan product in development, according to the FDA, is provided in Figure 5.2.

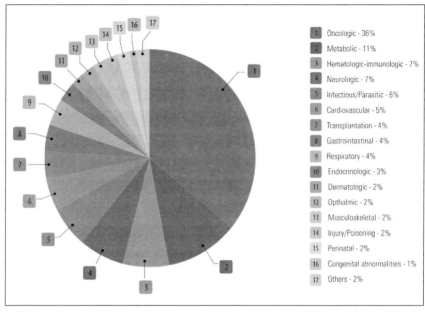

Figure 5.2. Disease categories targeted by Designated Orphan Drugs as a percentage of total (FDA data 2000 - 2006).

When I was a practicing family doctor, every year there would be a small number of cases amongst my 3,000 patients who either suffered some strange disease, or who joined my list with some pre-existing, but undiagnosed condition. In retrospect, I wonder how many of those often puzzling and frustrating cases (for the patient, their family and me) would now be diagnosable with modern gene sequencing technology.

NORD

In the decade before 1983, only ten new drugs were developed by industry for rare diseases. Since they affected no more than 200,000 Americans, they were receiving little attention. Research dollars and expertise were focused on the development of blockbuster drugs (see Chapter 1) for common diseases that were more likely to repay the huge costs of developing them. In 2010, it was estimated from publicly available data, that the cost to develop a new drug would exceed an astonishing one billion dollars.

Back in the early 1980s, leaders of rare disease patient advocacy organizations recognized that there were certain problems their patients with any rare disease and their families shared. It was clear that, while each disease may be rare, together these diseases affect millions of Americans, an estimated one in ten (probably thirty million patients). As a result, they collectively campaigned, calling for national legislation to encourage the development of treatments for rare diseases. The result was the 1983 ODA, and the patient advocacy leaders who had brought national recognition to the problem founded the National Organization for Rare Disorders (NORD) as an umbrella organization to represent the rare disease community.

NORD, a charitable organization, is a unique federation of over 130 voluntary health organizations that is committed to the identification, treatment, and cure of rare disorders through programs of education, advocacy, research, and service.

In theory, many rare genetically determined diseases that have previously been untreatable may now be amenable to one or more of the oligomers either in clinical development or in early preclinical development – or even in still earlier research.

There are numerous examples of oligomers already now in the clinical phase of their development for rare disease, i.e. they are now being tested in humans. The diseases for which they are targeted are provided in Figure 5.3. An update on these various programs and many other more common disease programs was provided by the sponsoring companies at a U.S. meeting hosted by the FDA and the Drug Information Association in April 2012.

Company	Oligomer	Rare Disease (Incidence/No. affected U.S.)	Status (see Chapter 9)
Isis	ATL1103	Acromegaly (3 per million/816 in U.S.)	Completed phase 1
Isis	ISIS-TTR$_{Rx}$	Hereditary Transthyretin Amyloidosis (50,000 patients worldwide)	Completed phase 1
Isis	ISIS-SOD1$_{Rx}$	Amyotrophic Lateral Sclerosis (ALS) (2 in 100,000)	In phase 1
Isis	ISIS-SMN$_{Rx}$	Spinal Muscular Atrophy (SMA) (1 in 10,000)	In phase 1
Alnylam*	ALN-TTR01/02	Hereditary Transthyretin Amyloidosis (50,000 patients worldwide)	In phase 2
Quark	QPI-1007	Non-arteritic ischemic optic neuropathy (1 in 200,000)	In phase 1
Antisense Pharma	Trabedersen	Glioma (cancer of the brain) (7 in 100,000)	In phase 2
Prosensa	PRO-051	Duchenne Muscular Dystrophy (exon 51) (13% of the 1 in 3,500 boys/ About 2,000)	In phase 3
Prosensa	PRO-044	Duchenne Muscular Dystrophy (exon 44) (6% of the 1 in 3,500 boys/ About 1,000)	In phase 2
AVI (now Sarepta)	Eteplirsen	Duchenne Muscular Dystrophy (exon 51) (13% of the 1 in 3,500 boys/ About 2,000)	In phase 2

* as of October 2012, Alnylam has partnered with Genzyme to develop this drug for Japanese and Asia-Pacific markets.

Figure 5.3 Oligomers currently in clinical development for rare disease indications

The companies developing new drugs for rare diseases benefit from the advocacy and various services NORD (and its European and Canadian counterparts) provides aimed at complementing them:

- Information about diseases and referrals to patient organizations (through their website at: http://www.rarediseases.org/rare-disease-information/rare-diseases)
- Patient assistance programs: Since 1987, NORD has helped patients receive drugs that could save or sustain their life. They also help with the cost of insurance, co-payment fees, diagnostic tests and even travel expenses so patients can see doctors who specialize in a particular rare disease.
- Research grants and fellowships
- Advocacy on public policy issues
- Help in forming organizations and mentoring for patient advocacy groups

NORD in July 2011 had information about 15 clinical studies on its website, for such diverse rare conditions as: Craniosynostosis (in California), Ehlers-Danlos Syndrome Type IV (EDS type IV) (in Washington), Hirschsprung Disease (at Johns Hopkins University) and Wegener's Granulomatosis (in Toronto, Canada). In addition, NORD produces regular newsletters for patients and their families and continues to stimulate congressional focus on addressing these previously underserved voters.

Whether due to the efforts of NORD or not, the general public has become more aware of these rare diseases.

EURORDIS

EURORDIS can be considered as the European equivalent of NORD, as a non-governmental patient-driven alliance representing more than 479 rare disease patient organizations in over 45 European countries, which was conceived for similar reasons. Founded in 1997, it is now administered by 26 staff based in Paris and Brussels. At the end of August 2010, EURORDIS settled into newly renovated dwellings in the grounds of the Hospital Broussais, Paris with their partners in the Plateforme Maladies Rares (Rare Diseases Platform) created in 2001. EURORDIS presents patient stories for 15 rare diseases (Alkaptonuria; Angelman syndrome; Chromosome 18 syndrome; Fragile X syndrome; Hereditary spastic paraplegia; Lysosomal disorders; Marfan syndrome; Marshall-Smith syndrome; Niemann-Pick; Osteogenesis imperfecta; Progeria; Retinitis pigmentosa; Spina bifida; Stiff man syndrome and Strumpell-Lorrain) on their website: http://www.eurordis.org/living-with-a-rare-disease.

EURORDIS has campaigned vigorously in Europe and claims to have made considerable progress. From their website (www.eurordis.org):

> ➢ EURORDIS assisted development and adoption of the EU regulation on Orphan Medicinal Products in 1999.
> ➢ EURORDIS participates in the Committee for Orphan Medicinal Products (COMP) at the EMA with two full members and one observer in the COMP. It thus plays an important role in the orphan drug development process in Europe.
> ➢ EURORDIS campaigned for incentives in the development of orphan drugs:
>> ➢ Fee waiver for orphan designation.
>> ➢ Reduced fees for Marketing Authorization Applications (the European equivalent for NDA), inspections, variations and protocol assistance.
>> ➢ Two year extension of market exclusivity for orphan pediatric drugs.

➢ EURORDIS currently advocates for:

> ➢ Parallel E.U.-U.S. submission and designation of orphan drugs to speed up development and access to new drugs based on a single regulatory submission.

> ➢ Creation of a Clinical Research Program for orphan drugs in support of designated products.

> ➢ National incentives such as research grants and tax credits.

➢ EURORDIS collaborates closely with the EMA for the production of quality information on orphan drugs for patients:

> ➢ At the time of orphan drug designation, EURORDIS reviews all Public Summaries of COMP opinion and liaises with concerned patient groups.

> ➢ At the time of marketing authorization, EURORDIS facilitates the reviewing of EPARs (European Public Assessment Reports) by patients with rare diseases.

➢ EURORDIS identifies and supports patient representatives to participate in:

> ➢ Protocol development assistance.

> ➢ Meetings of the scientific advice working party.

> ➢ Other meetings e.g. discussions on guidelines and risk management programs.

➢ EURORDIS has assisted over sixty rare disease patients provide input to the various orphan drug development process activities.

➢ EURORDIS advocates for patient access to authorized orphan drugs

> ➢ Regular surveys to assess and compare orphan drugs availability.

> ➢ Promotes European common policy and criteria for orphan drug access.

➢ EURORDIS Orphan Drug Task Force providing regular information updates to a network of volunteers affected by rare diseases:

   ➢ Two million EU citizens potentially benefitting from these drugs.

   ➢ 560 orphan drugs designated since 2000.

   ➢ 52 orphan drugs with marketing authorization in EU since 2000.

CORD

The Canadian Organization for Rare Disorders (CORD) is the national network of organizations that represents people affected by rare disorders within Canada. CORD's intention is to provide a strong common voice advocating for a healthcare system and health policy for those with rare disorders. Other countries are following the examples of the U.S., Canada and Europe and are also considering methods for encouraging development of orphan products, but with increasing harmonization, especially pertinent for orphan drugs, most national regulatory authorities tend to follow the lead of the FDA, EMA and PMDA.

In February 2008, the first Rare Disease Day was held in both Canada and Europe. The idea behind this holiday is to focus more attention on rare diseases. It has spread to the U. S. and takes place on February 28th each year, except leap years where it is observed on the 29th.

As a family doctor, I have served families who have had to deal with the diagnosis and management of a rare disease in their midst, and have had the experience myself. It is a life-changing experience. I am confident that the pharmaceutical industry is now on the road, with oligomers, to develop many novel drugs that will make enormous differences to the lives of patients afflicted with one of several rare diseases in the imminent future. If all goes well, as I think it will, the early oligomer approvals should herald the dawn of a new age in how medicines are discovered, designed and developed and we will truly see personalized medicine become a 21st century reality, and at last some hope for those 350 million people worldwide who suffer from a "rare" disease. So how do these oligomers treat rare disease? And do they cure the patients?

The answer to the second question is sadly, no. In the case of genetically determined disease, such as Duchenne muscular dystrophy (DMD), if your son has the genetic mutation it will be present throughout his life. However, by camouflaging that mutation using a very precisely targeted oligomer to bind to a short section of the pre-mRNA as it enters the nuclear spliceosome, it may be possible to splice out a mutant exon and splice together normal exons. Or the reading frame could be restored to allow a shorter but functional strand of mRNA to produce a shorter but functioning protein. In the case of DMD, that protein is dystrophin. Any splice switching or splice modulating oligomer will need to be taken for the rest of the patient's life to ensure that the same molecular gymnastics continue to occur for a happier and healthier future.

DMD is an example of how much more complex the story really is. Remember that there are 79 exons in the dystrophin gene. Any one of these, or more than one, may be missing or contain a mutation. Over the last thirty or so years, most boys with DMD are tested at diagnosis and the exact number and location of missing or mutated exons is determined. The data has been stored anonymously on a worldwide register. Doctors who diagnose a DMD child are encouraged to add details of every new case.

Leiden University in the Netherlands is where this database of genetic mutations for DMD is stored and overseen – and by 2006 over 4,600 different mutations of the dystrophin gene had been reported. Most of these led to either the severe DMD (if no dystrophin was produced as a result of the mutation), or the much milder Becker muscular dystrophy (BMD) if a shortened version of dystrophin was produced. In the latter situation, the mRNA might miss one or more exons but the sequence of three letter words was otherwise preserved and the mutation was said to be "in frame," allowing the ribosome to read the mature mRNA.

The difference between in frame and out of frame deletions can be explained using a sentence that I previously used, made up of three letter words to represent codons:

> ➢ *the big red fox ran far and saw the dog and cat hit the man*

An example of an out of frame deletion is where the last nucleotide from the second codon, the g of big is missing. After splicing the pre-mRNA exons together to form the mature mRNA, the message would read like this:

> ➢ *the bir edf oxr anf ara nds awt hed oga ndc ath itt hem an*

The ribosome would make no sense of this. Or maybe it might lead to the generation of an unwanted disease-causing protein. In the case of a boy with DMD, the vital dystrophin protein would be missing from the muscle cells. In the case of BMD, a whole codon or even several complete codons could be missing, for instance: "ran far and" but the remaining words in the message would still be intelligible. Although the sentence is short, and hence the sequence of amino acids in the finished dystrophin would be shorter than normal, the sentence still makes sense and the generated protein still works.

This is how a BMD in frame deletion mRNA message might read, using the above example:

> ➤ *the big red fox saw the dog and cat hit the man*

BMD patients may lead a completely normal active life and never even be diagnosed. Often, a diagnosis only occurs when they are being investigated for something else entirely.

The Leiden database stores the exact sequence, when it is known, for the many possible mutations, and allows researchers to determine which extra exon needs to be skipped, and in how many people, to potentially convert an out of frame mutation back into frame. In so doing, the idea is to convert the lethal DMD disease into a milder BMD. That hypothesis is now being actively tested in clinical studies in the U.S. and Europe, with encouraging preliminary results.

The database compares the sequence of codons for the same gene in different species – for instance it lists 46 vertebrates that have been so sequenced. This helps to know if the human disease has animal equivalents to test the oligomers on before going in to human studies. Three breeds of dogs – Labradors, Beagles and King Charles Spaniels have been discovered to have the canine equivalent of DMD. These unfortunate animals may help us with the development of oligomers for the human disease. In the case of the spaniels, the disease is very similar to the human one. It is lethal and only seen in male dogs. It is also genetically similar to the human disease and may be corrected by skipping exon 51 (of the 79 canine dystrophin exons). Skipping this exon to restore the reading frame is also the most common target in humans. The disease in beagles is due to a different mutation, still in the dystrophin gene, but in a different place. Beagles require a cocktail of three oligomers to overcome the mutation and restore the reading frame.

Scientists in Japan tested the three oligomer cocktail on some dystrophic beagles and the results, in comparison to an untreated littermate, even after only five weeks of therapy, were most encouraging.

These results can be seen in a pair of video clips on YouTube:

Untreated dog:

http://www.youtube.com/watch?v=lRzBc3kvhKM

Treated littermate:

http://www.youtube.com/watch?v=14VcMtpympI

Those of us who have worked in DMD, or in any of the other lethal rare diseases, always hope that this promising outcome can be replicated in humans and that the oligomer can be quickly made available.

However, there are many more steps that a new drug has to go through before that can happen. Two companies are already collaborating in large scale clinical studies testing the effectiveness and safety of their exon 51 skipping oligomer: the Dutch company Prosensa and the British pharmaceutical giant, GlaxoSmithKline. Not far behind is the U.S.'s Sarepta Therapeutics (formerly AVI BioPharma), with a different chemical class of oligomer. It's going through a longer, second study in DMD boys at a higher dose than was previously studied in the UK. In October 2012 Sarepta announced clinical benefits had been observed at 48 weeks in their study, and by December another announcement reported continued benefit seen at 62 weeks of dosing. There are high hopes that one or both programs will ultimately succeed and start to turn the tide on this dreadful disease.

When that day comes, it is very likely that more investment will flood into companies with promising oligomer candidates for other rare diseases. As the regulatory path for these promising treatments become familiar, the development of many other therapeutic oligomers becomes more feasible.

Of course, rare disease is only one area of the many potential uses of these oligomer-based drugs. Next I'll show you how they can destroy contagions and put an end to the spread of plague-like viruses.

Summary

Rare diseases affect one in every ten people worldwide. As the understanding of the human genome evolves, many more of the uncharacterized orphan diseases will become better understood and the exact genetic mutation leading to them documented. The opportunity to develop nucleic acid-based oligomers to treat these rare genetic mutations may become available. For some of these, research is now well underway; in a few examples, it has already entered the long awaited clinical studies. Hence the splice switching or translation suppressing oligomers may become real therapeutic options within the next few years.

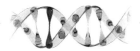

Chapter Six

New Drugs for Bad Bugs

R arely a week goes by without an alarming story of a new infectious agent ready to pounce on the unsuspecting public. The threat posed by bacteria becoming increasingly resistant to all the antibiotics we have developed is causing great concern within the medical and public health establishments. Rare but lethal viruses have emerged, probably crossing from animals to humans in Africa in the late 20th century. But where do all these bugs, both bacteria and viruses come from?

A recently completed project, the Human Microbiome Project, run by a consortium of scientists and overseen by the National Institutes of Health, checked out the microbiological flora from 242 adults over a period of 22 months. They published their results in a series of 16 papers. There were roughly 4,000 different bugs in the human gut that have a vital role in helping to break down food into more easily absorbed nutrients – with great diversity within each individual. For instance, there is a much greater variation between the organisms found in your nose, those found in your gut, or on your skin than there is between your gut flora and mine.

It has been estimated that there are roughly ten times the number of microbes living on or in you than the number of human cells in your body. And the number of bacterial genes you carry around is approximately one hundred times the number of your own genes. So we all live with these organisms in a healthy symbiosis.

However when you become ill, or acquire an infection, or destroy your healthy bacteria with a course of antibiotics, you create an open invitation for less helpful bugs to move in. Some of the most resistant bacteria are found lurking in hospitals where they have often acquired resistance to some, most or all of the available antibiotics. Getting an infection at a hospital can be lethal.

Bacteria

Bacteria are a large collection of single-celled, microorganisms. Typically a few micrometers in length, bacteria have a wide range of shapes, ranging from spheres (usually called cocci) to rods and spirals. Bacteria are ubiquitous in every habitat on earth, growing in soil, acidic hot springs, radioactive waste, water, and deep in the earth's crust, as well as in organic matter and the live bodies of plants and animals. They do not have a cell nucleus (karyon), and so are called "prokaryotes". Neither do they have any other membrane-bound organelles such as mitochondria, which are responsible for turning stored sugar into energy.

They do, however, have DNA and genes, usually in one chromosome, but not enclosed in a nucleus within the cell. This chromosome may contain up to several million base pairs, the bacterial genome. The human genome by comparison contains 3.1 billion base pairs but is not the largest genome yet discovered.

Organisms that have a cell nucleus are called eukaryotes, such as most of the animal and plant kingdoms. Unlike viruses, bacteria can grow and reproduce outside a host and are grown, for instance, on agar plates in laboratories, which is helpful when it comes to identifying them and testing for their susceptibility to antibiotics.

In a pinch of soil there are forty million bacteria. In a single drop of fresh water there are a million bacteria. Bacteria are extremely plentiful with an estimated five nonillion on planet Earth. That is five with 30 zeros after it! According to experts, the total mass of bacteria is greater than the combined weight of all animals and plants put together.

But bacteria are not all bad. They perform a valuable role in recycling nutrients, both in the soil and our guts. In fact digestion in many animals relies on intestinal bacteria. Bacteria also capture atmospheric nitrogen and help plants incorporate it and return nutrients from dead animals to the soil in the process of putrefaction. At least one example of half of the bacterial families can be grown. We remain woefully ignorant about the families of microbes in the half that we haven't been able to grow. Bacteriologists, the subset of microbiologists who study bacteria, are aiming to change that.

The vast majority of the bacteria in the body are harmless, as the body is protected by the immune system, and a few are even beneficial. However, certain species of bacteria are pathogenic and cause infectious diseases, which have haunted society over the millennia. Some cause massive outbreaks or epidemics, including cholera and bubonic plague. Others are spread by sexual contact with an infected person such as syphilis or carried in the air, like anthrax spores. Ironically, my late father, Professor John F. D. Shrewsbury (1898 – 1971) was a physician, bacteriologist, and medical historian who collected research material and wrote the seminal work on the history of the bubonic plague in the British Isles. He would have been fascinated, but likely not surprised, by the ongoing battle between bacteria and antibiotics.

In medieval Europe, tuberculosis (TB), or consumption, was responsible for many deaths. The organism gets into the lungs and slowly destroys the lung tissue. It has been beaten back largely in developed countries, although patients with immune disorders, AIDS, and other chronic diseases can still be susceptible. But in other parts of the world, sub-Saharan Africa for instance, TB is still rampant, with two million deaths per year. Respiratory infections in general are the leading infectious cause of death. The bugs are spread by coughing and sneezing which sends the bacteria into an invisible airborne mist, ready to be inhaled by the next victim.

Antibiotics cure many of the infections resulting from airborne bacterial attack, but they have been greatly overused. Physicians prescribe antibiotics too often when patients have viral diseases against which antibiotics are completely ineffective. In addition, antibiotics have been injudiciously used in agriculture, supplementing animal feed. Due to these two practices, antibiotic resistance has become common. There is now a growing organic movement that resists feeding free roaming animals these antibiotics. And doctors are strongly encouraged to be more thoughtful when considering whether to prescribe one.

But bacteria do have their uses. Sewage treatment utilizes them. At the other end of the gastrointestinal tract, so does the food industry. Bacteria are used to ferment milk to generate yogurt and cheese. Lastly, in an ironic twist, some bacteria have been tamed by the biotechnology industry and are used to manufacture antibiotics and other biological drugs.

Bacteria were first observed by Antonie van Leeuwenhoek in 1676 using a single-lens microscope of his own design. Van Leeuwenhoek (1632–1723) lived in Delft in the Netherlands. His greatest contribution to science was his work on the improvement of the microscope. Using his rudimentary, handcrafted microscopes, Van Leewenhoek was the first to observe small, single celled microbes which he called *animalcules*. He wrote up his observations in a series of letters to the Royal Society. Van Leewenhoek was also the first to observe muscle fibers, spermatozoa and blood flow in capillaries (small blood vessels). The term *"bacterium"* was introduced much later, by Christian Gottfried Ehrenberg, in 1828.

One important and well-known figure in the study of bacteria was Louis Pasteur (1822 – 1895). He was a French chemist and physicist, becoming a professor in both sciences before focusing on microbiology after three of his five children died of typhoid fever. He did remarkable pioneering work on the causes and preventions of illnesses, establishing the germ theory of disease, supported by his experimental data. His discoveries reduced mortality from puerperal fever, and he created the first vaccine for rabies and anthrax.

Pasteur is best known to the general public for inventing a method to stop milk and wine from causing sickness, a process that came to be called pasteurization.

Another early bacteriologist of renown was Robert Koch (1843 – 1910), a German physician, who with Pasteur was an early advocate of the germ theory of disease. In his research into tuberculosis, Koch finally proved the germ theory, for which he was awarded a Nobel Prize in 1905. In *Koch's postulates*, he set out criteria to test if an organism is the cause of a disease, and these postulates are still used today.

Though it was known in the nineteenth century that bacteria are the cause of many diseases, no effective antibacterial treatments were available. Paul Ehrlich (1854 – 1915) was another German physician who became interested in staining cells and bacteria and looking at them under the microscope. He attracted attention and was invited to join Koch at the Institute of Infectious Disease in Berlin in 1891. In 1910, Ehrlich developed the first antibiotic, by changing dyes that selectively stained *Treponema pallidum*, the spirochete that causes syphilis, into compounds that selectively killed the pathogen. Ehrlich had been awarded a Nobel Prize in 1908 for his work on immunology, and pioneered the use of stains (such as Gram stain) to detect and identify bacteria.

However, let us skip forward one hundred years to today. Why are pathogenic (disease causing) bacteria a problem when, following on from penicillin, there are now multiple classes of antibiotics? Surely there are enough antibiotics to treat every bacterial infection. Indeed there are over twenty classes of antibiotics.

With so many different classes of antibiotics, how is it that some bacteria remain almost impossible to treat?

The main reason is that bacteria replicate very quickly and with each generation genetic mutations can occur. Some of those mutations will lead to weaker bugs, and they will die off. Some bacteria will have no mutation and they will be killed off by the antibiotic to which they were formerly susceptible. But if even a very few bacteria develop a mutation conferring resistance to the chosen antibiotic, this new colony will very quickly multiply.

Bacterial populations can double in size in less than ten minutes! That means in one hour a single resistant bacterium could have become 64, by two hours 4096. In just 24 hours, that single bacterium could easily spawn 2.23×10^{43} offspring!

Over the last fifty years, since antibiotics became available, they have tended to be vastly overused, often prescribed for viral infections which do not respond to antibiotics, which has allowed some harmless bacteria (and some harmful ones) to be exposed to low levels of the antibiotic. In addition antibiotics have been added to animal feeds and by eating the meat from animals from these intensively farmed livestock, humans have been chronically exposed to low levels of antibiotics. This "encourages" the bacteria to develop resistance genes which can be transferred between bacteria in a horizontal fashion by conjugation, transduction, or transformation. Thus a gene for antibiotic resistance that has evolved via natural selection may be shared. Evolutionary stress such as exposure to antibiotics then selects for the antibiotic resistant trait. If a bacterium carries several resistance genes, it is called multi-resistant or, informally, a superbug or super bacterium, of which Methicillin-resistant *Staphylococcus Aureus* (MRSA), Vancomycin-resistant Enterococci (VRE) and Fluoroquinolone-resistant *Pseudomonas aeruginosa* (FQRP) are feared examples (Figure 6.1).

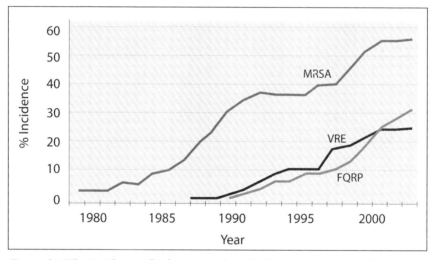

Figure 6.1. The incidence of infection by three highly resistant bacterial organisms (Methicillin-resistant *Staphylococcus* Aureus [MRSA], Vancomycin-resistant Enterococci [VRE] and Fluoroquinolone-resistant *Pseudomonas aeruginosa* FQRP]) over the last thirty years in the U.S. (Source CDC)

The longer you are exposed to an antibiotic; the greater your risk of developing resistant bugs, irrespective of the severity of your infection. As resistance towards antibiotics becomes more common, a greater need for alternative treatments arises. However, despite a push for new antibiotic therapies, there has been a continued decline in the number of newly approved drugs. Indeed the Infectious Disease Society of America – the professional body representing ID doctors – has urged in its "Bad Bugs Need Drugs" campaign for ten new antibiotics to be developed by 2020. It was the IDSA who coined the phrase "Bad Bugs, No Drugs" in 2004 when they raised concerns about the stagnation of antibiotic discovery and development (Figure 6.2), claiming it was a public health crisis.

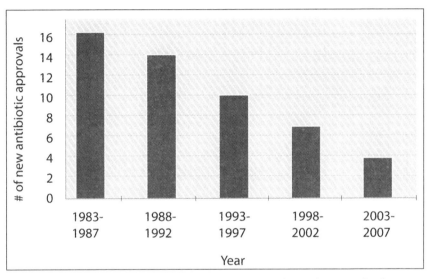

Figure 6.2. Total number of new antibiotic approvals in the U.S. for five year periods over 25 years. (After Spellberg et al., CID January, 2009:48)

Of special concern to the IDSA and healthcare in general are the so-called ESKAPE organisms – *enterococcus faecium, staphylococcus aureus, klebsiella pneumoniae, acinetobacter baumanii, pseudomonas aeruginosa,* and *enterobacter* species. Just their names are scary enough. These six bacteria are currently the cause of most U.S. hospital acquired infections. The staphylococcus is MRSA. Due to their high resistance they "escape" the infection control and antibacterial efforts of the institution. Nearly every week an outbreak of infection by one or more of these ESKAPE superbugs is reported somewhere in the U.S.

The number of reports is steadily climbing, with more states finding them (Figure 6.3).

But the U.S. is not alone (Figure 6.4). The scientific literature is also being showered with reports of resistance genes, often carried on plasmids (which are small round bundles of DNA within bacteria but separate from the chromosome), which can be exchanged between bacteria passing on resistance.

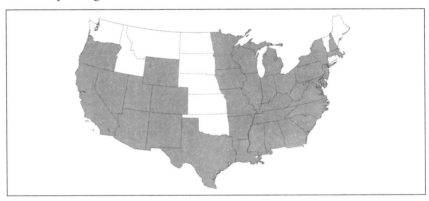

Figure 6.3. Location of Carbapenem-Resistant *Enterobacteriaceae* (CRE) in the United Sates caused by Klebsiella pneumonia carbapenemase enzyme

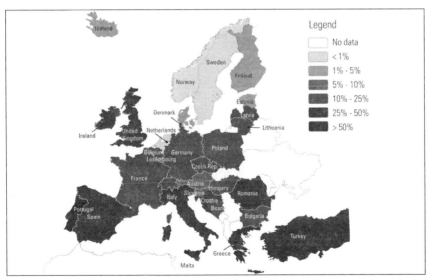

Figure 6.4. Incidence of MRSA in human blood samples in a 2008 European study.

Hospitals the world over keep careful records of the number of patients who acquire an infection during an admission, and these statistics have been used to help shape and monitor important infection control policies. In the UK, the number of deaths due to hospital acquired MRSA or *Clostridium difficile* were 364 and 2053 respectively in 2011. The deaths due to *C. difficile* represented one percent of all hospital deaths, so despite a small reduction in 2010 deaths, there is no room for complacency.

Emerging resistance to antibiotics is not confined to the fast growing bacteria however. Tuberculosis is a slower growing bacterium, making it challenging to grow in the laboratory and to determine its profile of sensitivity, or resistance, to antibiotics. To treat it successfully usually requires a combination of up to four different drugs, for several months, to ensure that as the bug becomes resistant to one or more antibiotics, as it invariably does, it will still be susceptible to at least one other.

Tuberculosis used to be very prevalent in the western world, but over the last one hundred years, increasingly sophisticated treatment has greatly reduced, but not eliminated, the disease from America and Europe. However other countries have not had similar success. India, like many of the countries in sub-Saharan Africa, has two million new cases of TB every year, with one thousand deaths every single day due to the disease. More concerning is the emergence of a strain of TB that is resistant to most of today's drugs, so called multi-drug resistance TB (MDR-TB). To make matters worse, new strains are emerging that appear to be resistant to every antibiotic, making them untreatable. This former scourge of medieval Europe could be about to make a comeback and we are woefully ill equipped to tackle it.

As science has become more sophisticated, dramatically so in the last few decades, so we have become better equipped to track where these multi-drug resistant bacteria are, and in many cases, how they got there. Using gene sequencing technology we are able to identify the resistance genes they have acquired, and how they acquired them by mutation or from plasmid exchange from another organism.

In addition we have identified the vital proteins that these bacterial genes produce, and, importantly, the sequence of nucleotides in the gene (and hence in the mRNA) necessary for generating each of those proteins. Some of these nucleotide sequences are identical between different bacterial species.

The next step is to take this knowledge and build oligomers against those sequences and use them as "antibiotics." Why hasn't this been done? Actually it has. With good results, although this application is really in its infancy. As a scientific paper entitled "Antisense antibiotics: a brief review of novel target discovery and delivery" by Bai and colleagues published in *Current Drug Discovery Technology* in June 2010 puts it, "The concept of using antisense antibiotics has experienced ups and downs in the past decade. In the past five years, however, significant technology advances in the fields of microbial genomics, structural modification of oligonucleotides and efficient delivery system have led to fundamental progress in the research and in vivo application of this paradigm. The wealthy information provided in the microbial genomics era has allowed the identification and/or validation of a number of essential genes that may serve as possible targets for antisense inhibition."

An interesting fact about this article is that the six authors are all from the School of Pharmacy at the Military University in X'ian, China. Maybe the next wave of new, effective antibiotics, oligomers, will come from Asia? Actually, although there are currently no clinical studies registered for antibacterial oligomers on ClinicalTrials.Gov, AVI BioPharma, now Sarepta Therapeutics, and possibly other companies working with PMOs, as well as companies with other oligomers, have preliminary laboratory data against several of the "bad (bacterial) bugs." This data suggests that although there are no drugs currently marketed, there are options in early development.

PMO stands for phosphorodiamidate morpholino oligomer, a particular charge-neutral chemistry which Sarepta pioneered and has been working on for close to thirty years. Indeed Sarepta, based now in Bothell, Washington (Figure 2.1, #12) is the oldest of the small band of oligonucleotide companies.

One of Sarepta's collaborating scientists from Oregon State University as far back as 2005 reported in *Current Opinions in Molecular Therapy* that shorter oligomers that are ten to twenty units in length, whether with or without a membrane-permeating peptide attached, should be effective against *Escherichia coli*, *Staphylococcus aureus* and *Mycobacterium tuberculosis* (TB). In addition, Sarepta has published early animal data showing that one of their oligomers against *Burkholderia cepacia* (another nasty, currently untreatable bug that can infect the airways of patients with cystic fibrosis) and *Bacillus anthracis* (anthrax) is effective. In 2011, Sarepta announced a timely collaboration with the prestigious Swedish Karolinska Institute to identify oligomers to treat extensively drug-resistant TB (XDR-TB).

There is much work to be done before any of these new antibacterial translation-suppressing oligomers (TSOs) can start being tested in healthy human volunteers, let alone being tried on infected patients in controlled clinical trials. But it seems likely that either PMOs alone or mixed with various other oligomers could be developed against many of these scary bacteria in the next decade. This is reassuring to know, as resistance to current antibiotics is sure to increase.

An extra benefit of using these TSOs is that resistance will not develop to them. They block production of essential proteins made by the bacteria. There does not appear to be a work-around solution that the bacteria can use to avoid these novel antibacterial agents. By targeting the mRNA from the bacterial gene, these oligomers tackle the issue at the root cause.

Viruses

In 1898, Friedrich Loeffler (1852 – 1915), who had also worked with Koch in Berlin, and Paul Frosch (1860 – 1928), recognized that the cause of foot-and-mouth disease in livestock was an infectious particle smaller than any bacteria. This was the first clue to the nature of viruses, genetic entities that lie somewhere in the grey area between living and non-living states.

Viruses are very simple structures. They cannot reproduce outside of their host's cells. Unlike bacteria, they cannot be grown on an agar plate. They can be grown in the laboratory in living cells – a tissue culture. In fact viruses have to hijack their host's cellular machinery to reproduce. Viruses depend on the host cells that they infect to reproduce, and unlike bacteria, cannot reproduce outside of their host's cells. They can, however, survive outside of host cells. In those cases, they exist as a protein coat or capsid, sometimes enclosed within a membrane. The capsid encloses either DNA or RNA that codes for the viral protein elements. When found as a capsid, the virus is metabolically inert, as if it's in suspended animation, Sleeping Beauty if you will. Once inside a host, it becomes active.

When a host cell is exposed to a virus, the virus can insert its genetic material into its host, literally taking over the host's cellular functions. An infected cell produces more viral protein and genetic material instead of its usual products. The cell's protein making functions are literally hijacked by the virus.

There are many viruses. Indeed, keeping up with the new viruses as they are discovered and classified is challenging. The International

Committee on Taxonomy of Viruses describes six orders (groupings) each with three to five families and then 65 families not assigned to an order. The families are then split into genera – much the same system of naming as seen with animals and plants.

Why is this relevant?

Knowing how a virus is related to other viruses may help us understand them better and lead to antiviral therapies sooner. Several closely related viruses may possibly be susceptible to the same therapeutic agent. For oligomers, the RNA viruses are important. As they release their viral RNA into a cell, oligomers can be made that recognize specific viral RNA. This may permit the blocking of that viral RNA from translating the proteins it requires in the cell's ribosomes. These new oligomers are therefore called "translation suppressing oligomers" (TSOs).

There are several types of RNA viruses. Two examples are single-stranded RNA (ssRNA) and double-stranded RNA (dsRNA). Several important human diseases are caused by RNA viruses, including SARS, influenza, hepatitis C, Ebola and Marburg Hemorrhagic Fevers.

RNA viruses can be further classified according to the "sense" or polarity of their RNA into negative-sense and positive-sense RNA viruses. Positive-sense viral RNA is similar to the host cell mRNA and thus can be immediately translated by the ribosomes of the host cell. Negative-sense viral RNA is complementary to mRNA and must be converted to positive-sense RNA first by an RNA polymerase before translation.

The double-stranded (ds) RNA viruses represent a diverse group of viruses that vary widely in host range (humans, animals, plants, fungi, and bacteria), genome segment number (one to twelve), and virion organization (e.g. the number of capsid layers).

Viral RNA is of the same design, with the same 4 letters (A, C, G and U) as human mRNA. Recall RNA is the key molecule that has allowed there to be life on Earth, and all life shares the same building blocks. That is why a virus is able to hijack the host cell's ribosome and convert it to forming more viral proteins. The viral proteins are then packaged up and new viral particles are released as the host cell is overcome and dies.

The viral RNA, however, is so predictable and consistent that once the sequence of letters has been established, an oligomer can be quickly built to bind by Watson-Crick base pairing to the complementary sequence of viral RNA and prevent the ribosome from translating more viral protein.

Sarepta Therapeutics, has achieved the remarkable feat of designing and manufacturing sufficient quantities of oligomers to start animal testing against influenza (in 2010) and Dengue (in 2011) viruses in response to requests from the Department of Defense in seven and eleven days respectively. Normally the process of initial concept to small scale production of a drug takes several years, and involves many scientists, researchers and considerable financial support. But sequencing the letters in viral RNA is now rapid. Building a complementary oligomer is straightforward, cutting years off drug development timelines.

To design effective antiviral oligomers requires considerable experience, and a certain amount of educated guesswork. One has to pick the right viral gene to target and what part of the gene transcript to camouflage.

As noted above there are many classes of virus, many of which cause disease in humans and most of which do not have any specific treatment available. Prevention of viral disease has evolved greatly since the time of Edward Jenner, an English family doctor, who in 1796 first injected pus from a cowpox pustule to protect against the closely related, but often lethal smallpox virus.

Vaccination, which is what Jenner achieved, has effectively eradicated smallpox from the world. Other viruses, such as polio, seem destined to be eradicated too, or at least dramatically reduced by vaccination. These illnesses include measles, mumps, rubella (German measles) and some viruses that lead to cancer, such as Hepatitis B (which leads to hepatoma, liver cancer) or human papilloma virus (HPV, which leads to cervical cancer in women). The list continues to grow.

Other viruses that have recently emerged as dangerous to humans have started to attract increasing attention. Some of these viruses are thought to have jumped species from animal hosts where they may not be so lethal. Ebola and Marburg viruses are two such that are members of the filovirus family.

The U.S. Department of Defense is concerned lest a terrorist try to include one or more of the Hemorrhagic Fever viruses, Ebola or Marburg being the likeliest, into a weapon to be used in the U.S. Currently these viruses are being intensively studied in ultra-secure laboratories, but accidents happen and scientists working with these agents have received needle stick injuries several times. Oligomers have been developed to combat these agents and have been very effective in animals.

Filoviruses

In 1967, while many were enjoying the swinging sixties, an outbreak of a strange hemorrhagic fever swept through Marburg, a town in Germany. Spreading to other European locations, 37 patients were affected, and seven died. Investigating the cause, scientists discovered a new family of virus: the filoviridae family. The particular virus that caused the outbreak was isolated and named Marburg virus.

The reason monkeys were shipped from Africa to Marburg in Germany was to provide African monkeys as a source of fresh kidneys, which were used in the preparation of polio vaccine. Normally the animals were shipped from Uganda to Cairo, Egypt, where they were held in quarantine. In 1967, there was an incident at Entebbe airport in Uganda when a plane was hijacked, so on this occasion the shipment of monkeys was diverted direct to Marburg, unfortunately with a live Marburg virus incubating. Those infected had been exposed to blood or tissue from the monkeys, unaware that the deadly cargo of filoviridae was lurking in the monkey cells.

The Marburg virus is an enveloped, non-segmented, negative-stranded RNA virus. The infection it causes is zoonotic, meaning that the virus is transmitted to humans from other animals, possibly bats. The mechanisms through which filoviruses spread are not fully understood. The route of transmission from other animals to humans is unknown, although eating meat from infected monkeys has led to human cases. Person-to-person transmission occurs primarily through physical contact, making strict quarantine and barrier nursing essential in managing cases.

Most subsequent human outbreaks, since the original Marburg 1967 scare, have occurred in sub-Saharan Africa, of which 2,300 cases have been reported leading to 1,670 deaths, a high mortality rate.

In Western countries, Marburg hemorrhagic fever (MHF) can be transmitted through coming into contact with blood or other infected fluids. Though this disease rarely occurs, what makes it frightening is that as many as eighty percent of the patients who contract it die. Studies in animals have shown that it can be contracted via droplets. After the Ustinov incident Marburg seemed to disappear, but it reappeared twenty years later, in July of 2008. MHF was confirmed in a 41-year old Dutch woman who had returned from a vacation in Uganda. Exposure to the virus is thought to have occurred on a visit to a cave. The patient and two other tourists had visited the empty caves in Fort Portal with a guide, and the Python Cave, in Maramagambo Forest, a few days later. The caves were known to have colonies of bats living there. These bats had been found positive for Marburg virus elsewhere in Africa. The woman had complained about being sick with fever and chills for three days shortly after her return, and she was hospitalized on July 5th but not initially quarantined. By July 7th, her dramatically deteriorating condition prompted the concern that she had a hemorrhagic fever and she was transferred to a specialist quarantine unit at the Leiden University Medical Center in Holland.

Marburg filovirus infection was confirmed by the Bernard-Nocht-Institute for Tropical Medicine in Hamburg, Germany on July 10th, but with no treatment available, the woman died on July 11th. Although only one patient was confirmed with MHF, a response team was formed to monitor the crisis. In total, 130 contacts were identified (66 classified as high risk and 64 as low risk) and monitored for 21 days after their last possible exposure. The case raised questions specific to international travel, post-exposure prophylaxis for Marburg virus, and laboratory testing of contacts with fever.

The Ustinov Incident

In early April 1988, the director of a huge, isolated virology-research campus in the forests outside Novosibirsk, a city in western Siberia, reported that there had been an accident. At that time, the Soviet biological missile warheads were designed to be loaded with smallpox virus, Black Death, and anthrax. The Marburg virus had potential to be used as a weapon too.

Dr. Ustinov was 44 years old, and had been doing basic military research on the Marburg virus, studying its potential as a weapon. Ustinov was used to working in a special suit – more like an astronaut's spacesuit – and working in ultra secure conditions with strict quarantine. He spent his days injecting the lethal experimental

---

Marburg virus into guinea pigs and trying to learn how it behaved. On one occasion however he pricked his finger with the needle which went through both layers of rubber gloves. Ustinov immediately called his supervisor who decided that Ustinov should be admitted to a bio-containment hospital for observation. The facility had twenty beds, which could only be reached through steel air-lock doors, like the doors of a submarine. The nurses and doctors caring for Ustinov moved around in carefully sealed spacesuits, similar to the one Ustinov himself had been wearing.

Ustinov was not afraid of dying, but, he was not allowed to see his wife or children and he became deeply depressed. The waiting must have been terrible for all concerned and by day four he developed a headache. Then, tiny hemorrhages started to appear on the whites of his eyes. He started to make detailed notes of how he felt in a daily diary, as the space-suited medical staff worked to keep him alive. Soon Ustinov needed blood transfusions to replace blood lost through his gut. He had begun to vomit blood and pass bloody black diarrhea. But as the blood was pumped into his veins it came pouring out of his mouth and rectum. Ustinov's condition deteriorated rapidly as he developed star shaped hemorrhages in his skin. As he wrote his diary, blood oozed from his pores and a trail of bloody fingerprints smeared the pages.

On April 30, 1988, Ustinov died.

The second genus of the filoviridae family, Ebola virus, was discovered to be the cause of an outbreak in 1976 at Ngaliema Hospital in Kinshasa, in northern Zaire. A mortality rate of up to ninety percent has been reported in some Ebola outbreaks. The name comes from the Ebola River Valley in the Democratic Republic of the Congo (formerly

Zaire), which is near the site of the first recognized outbreak. It remained largely unheard of until 1989, when several widely publicized outbreaks occurred among monkeys in the U.S. The virus interferes with the cells lining the interior surface of blood vessels and with blood clotting. As the blood vessel walls become damaged and destroyed, the platelets are unable to coagulate, and patients bleed from every orifice, and even the skin, just as with Dr. Ustinov and his closely allied Marburg hemorrhagic fever. Ebola is transmitted through bodily fluids, while conjunctival exposure may also lead to transmission.

In 1989, an Ebola variant was found in a group of cynomolgus macaques at a facility in Reston, Virginia near Washington, D.C. This "Reston" strain was harmful to macaques but was not pathogenic to humans who were exposed. Infection patterns were consistent with possible airborne transmission. This terrifying but true story is told by Richard Preston in the book, *The Hot Zone*.

In 2009, an Ebola-Reston infection of pigs was reported. There is ongoing concern that the infection of swine could contaminate the food supply or lead to the emergence of an airborne Ebola variant that affects humans.

Both Ebola and Marburg are therefore frightening viruses to contemplate. They are not well understood. Their natural host(s) are not clearly defined. They are highly transmissible to humans from their natural hosts and once humans are infected, very high mortality rates are seen, leading to intensive quarantine precaution and barrier nursing of the highest level of rigor. Lastly, neither virus is treatable; there is only supportive care to give while the doctors and nurses watch the patients die (or in a few cases, recover) on their own.

The U.S. and other governments are very concerned about the possibility of a lethal, highly transmissible virus appearing and spreading as the planet becomes more crowded and international travel more available. This could become a replay of the 1918 Spanish Flu outbreak which in three successive waves over a short period (1918-1919) killed an estimated fifty to one hundred million people around the world.

Returning to the present day, another needle stick injury occurred at the Bernard-Nocht-Institute in Hamburg, Germany, to a scientist while working with the deadly Ebola virus in March 2009. Amid a flurry of activity in Germany and the U.S. (in which I was peripherally involved), I rapidly came to realize how urgent the need was for a safe and effective treatment to be developed for Ebola Hemorrhagic Fever before any more laboratory workers were accidentally infected, and before any further outbreaks occurred in the African jungle. In this latest incident the worker did not contract the infection.

Against the fictitious and factual outbreaks and incidents, there is currently no effective treatment for filovirus infections. But that situation may be about to change.

In July 2010, Sarepta Therapeutics announced that it had been awarded a contract worth up to $291 million by the U.S. Department of Defense to develop oligomers to counter the Ebola and Marburg virus infections. The contracts were to cover the scale up of manufacturing to large scale provision, the preclinical (animal) safety testing and additional efficacy studies in animals as well as all the clinical work, plans which I designed and wrote into the submission with the help of colleagues and consultants. Preliminary data for the efficacy of the translation suppressing oligomers for both Ebola and Marburg is very encouraging and has been presented at international scientific meetings. The results show that the oligomers can turn a one hundred percent fatality rate in monkeys inoculated with virus but without drug, to a sixty percent (Ebola) or one hundred percent (Marburg) survival rate with the addition of the oligomer.

The same oligomer should be suitable in humans if infected. Both programs already have successfully tested the different oligomers in humans for safety. They appear to be well tolerated under very carefully controlled observation; the doses were carefully increased to what is hoped to be a potentially effective dose.

Now that the Ebola and Marburg oligomers have passed this first important hurdle and appear to have acceptable safety profiles, there will be intense excitement as the development plans unfold.

The threat of bioterrorism remains of great concern more than a decade after 9/11. The subsequent successful but limited and unattributed anthrax attacks claimed five lives and injured 17. Project Bioshield was enacted by Congress in 2004 to try and address these terrifying bio-threats.

Much of the preparation for a possible future attack has been led by the Biomedical Advanced Research and Development Authority (BARDA), which has concentrated on the agents they predict as the most likely to be used. These are smallpox (a virus) and anthrax (a bacterium).

These agents are the top two on a list at the Department of Homeland Security that contains a total of twelve potentially threatening microbial agents: bacillus anthracis (anthrax), burkholderia mallei (glanders), burkholderia pseudomallei (melioidosis), clostridium botulinum (botulism), Ebola virus (hemorrhagic fever), francisella tularensis (tularemia), junin virus (hemorrhagic fever), Marburg virus (hemorrhagic fever), multidrug-resistant bacillus anthracis (MDR anthrax), rickettsia prowazekii (typhus), variola major (smallpox) and yersinia pestis (plague).

Progress is slow, despite an investment of twenty billion dollars. The National Biodefense Science Board, an independent panel of biodefense experts from industry, academia and government, reported in March 2010 that the U.S. Government had "failed to mobilize the productive skills and efforts of industry" ["Where Are the Counter-measures"]. A further report from the National Security Council, in November 2009, estimated that a successful bioterrorist plot could cost the country up to one trillion dollars for each incident.

In contrast, BARDA's director is confident that the U.S. biodefense effort will develop and procure medical countermeasures against the full range of probable bioterror pathogens within the next five years. Part of the problem has been the uncertainty about the provision of funds. These awards are often given much later than they are initially intended, keeping companies waiting while they continue to have to meet their staff payrolls. That situation is unsustainable for small biotech companies. But these same small companies are exactly the ones that have shown most interest in developing novel antiviral drugs or vaccines.

Recent estimates of drug development costs suggest they now exceed one billion dollars per drug and require ten years of work, according to the New York Times. Thus, if we wish to have a vaccine for each emerging agent, then we need forty new drugs. Do we really need to pay forty billion dollars and take four hundred cumulative years to accomplish this?

In addition, though there used to be a "guarantee" to small companies that development of a product against these otherwise rare infections, would lead to procurement, that guarantee has been removed. Small companies and their investors, are, therefore, reluctant to risk spending their resources on development with no guarantee they will recoup at some future point from BARDA.

Another challenge is how to develop these oligomers against a possible future bioterrorist attack. One of the mechanisms designed to encourage development of therapeutic agents against these infections, the "Animal Rule," has yet to be fully tested amid mixed messages from the FDA. The Office of Counter-Terrorism and Emerging Threats has been established by the FDA to try and smooth progress of novel agents through the increasingly complex regulatory system, but it and the CDER division responsible for review of any NDA do not always appear to be on the same page. In fact that changed in December 2012 with the FDA approving GSK's monoclonal antibody, raxibacumab, for inhalational anthrax. The biologic was developed by Human Genome Sciences and is the first drug approved by the "Animal Rule."

The "Animal Rule" is intended to offer an alternative way to establish efficacy data in infectious diseases where testing in humans would be unfeasible, unethical or both, which is the case with the twelve microbes identified above. However, for this rule to be applied, there needs to be a suitable animal model of the disease. This may be hard to identify and then demonstrate to the FDA's satisfaction.

Still, some progress has been made and over the next decade we will have a chance to see if these developments bear fruit.

But it is not only these twelve known microbes that raise the hair on the back of my neck. What about the simple influenza virus, if it changes to the deadly epidemic, Spanish Flu of 1918? Or if the H5N1 (bird flu) virus, that caused alarm and deaths a few years ago, comes back? Controversial research was published in 2012 by a team of scientists in the Netherlands, who identified that there would only need to be five changes to the H5N1 virus gene for it to become much more transmissible. It is another virus without any current effective remedy. Indeed, this real life scientific study is frightfully close to some of the elements of the plot of the movie *Contagion*, where an unknown infection spreads to millions of people in just a few days – before an antidote or cure is developed. It is worrying to think about what would happen in real life if a lethal virus acquired the transmissibility of a less dangerous, easily disseminated one. Other movies have glued viewers to their seats by dramatizing the likely effect of a rapidly spreading virus. In 1995, *Outbreak* featured a virus resembling Ebola, and two years later, the movie *Pandemic* was based on the bird flu H5N1 virus.

But you do not need to rent a movie to see how horrifying these viruses can be. In August 2012, an outbreak of Ebola struck an isolated village in the Kibaale district of western Uganda. Within a few days, 16 patients had died and surrounding communities saw panicked residents fleeing from the area. Television and newspaper coverage showed pictures of healthcare workers in space suits caring for the infected. They tried to isolate and contain the deadly, highly contagious virus in the absence of any effective treatment. So far the outbreak seems to have been contained, although whole families have been wiped out. Next time, or the time after that, will we be so lucky? Or will an outbreak hit the huge, densely crowded cities of America, Europe, Asia, Africa or Australia where it may be much harder to contain?

Summary

As the planet becomes increasingly crowded, new "bad bugs" emerge, both viral and bacterial. It is inevitable that there will be a delay before modern medicine comes up with a curative (or preventative) treatment against them. Many pharmaceutical companies have shied away from trying to develop new antibiotics. The costs for development have skyrocketed and the regulatory hurdles have become ever higher. Thus, the risk of new bugs emerging and spreading quickly in a devastating epidemic has become a great worry to public health officials and infectious disease doctors around the world. Media attention has fuelled public anxiety, as seen with the SARS outbreak and more recently, the swine flu. Both of these viral infections have slipped off the public radar for now, but remain very much on the minds of public health doctors and departments, and governments, too. The fear that an even more virulent bug, such as Ebola or Marburg virus may break out, either accidentally or intentionally triggered, keeps many scientists and doctors working tirelessly to develop countermeasures. Some oligomer-based drugs are now entering clinical trials in humans and primates. These oligomers will be "personalized" not just against a specific bug, but against the generation of a specific protein which may be shared with other bugs, making the translation suppressing oligomers appropriate for treating more than one of these bugs.

So although the status today is "Bad Bugs – No Drugs," tomorrow there may be new drugs that can block the messages coming from the microbe's genes that are responsible for their lethality in humans.

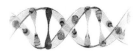

Chapter Seven

The Big Ones: Common, Chronic Diseases

Chronic and common diseases such as asthma, cancer and heart disease are scourges of modern life. Pharmacy shelves are filled with blockbuster drugs aimed at controlling the symptoms of these diseases. But, none of these drugs address the actual cause of these conditions. And, many come with significant side effects. Oligomers can target the root cause of disease, the message that each cell transmits from its genes to the protein-making machinery. By doing so they will prevent the disease from manifesting without harming you.

There are exciting developments in personalized medicine for treating breast, prostate and lung cancers, and leukemia. Taken together, these ailments claimed the lives of 666,970 Americans in 2011.

Genetics plays a part in a significant percentage of these diseases, and many of the responsible genes may be amenable to oligomer therapy. For example:

- There are approximately seventy genes listed on the Leukemia Gene Database related to twenty different leukemias.

- Most of the five to ten percent of breast and ovarian cancers that are believed to be inherited are linked to the well known BRCA1 and BRCA2 genes.
- In January of 2012, genes were identified for both prostate and lung cancer.

Oligomers also hold promise for the development of therapies for other common diseases such as asthma, high cholesterol, and arthritis. You're about to discover how oligomers can address some of the most prevalent diseases that either you, or someone you know may suffer from now or in the future.

On June 26, 2000, the first Human Genome was sequenced. President Bill Clinton truly recognized how momentous this event was " …this is the most important, most wondrous map ever produced by humankind," he said. "With this profound new knowledge, humankind is on the verge of gaining immense new power to heal. Genome science will have a real impact on ALL our lives, and even more, on the lives of our children. It will revolutionize the diagnosis, prevention, and treatment of most, if not all, human disease."

He was right. Nothing he said was an exaggeration. Here's why:

We appear to be close to exhausting the potential supply of (small molecule) drugs for all the potential targets of the "druggable" genome. We are also struggling to keep ahead of bacterial resistance and have had lamentable lack of success treating virus infections. So where are the next generation of therapies in medicine going to come from? And, just as important, can they tackle anything more than the rare genetic diseases or the lethal killer viruses which have by and large stayed away from the Northern Hemisphere's shores?

From the moment in 1978 when Harvard professor Paul Zamecnik performed his experiment with an oligonucleotide to demonstrate a blocking effect that was predictable, tremendous advances in research on how and when to manipulate RNA have been taking place. Over the same period, especially the last decade, there has been a worrying slump in the number of new (small molecule) drugs receiving approval. In addition those that have been approved have had to struggle with the rapid, dramatic and inexorable increase in development cost and time.

The interest in developing oligomers for rare diseases has occurred simultaneously with the mapping of the Human Genome. The two go together "hand in glove", and their time has now come for modern medicine to benefit from them.

Within the next twenty years many major diseases, the big ones, such as arthritis, coronary heart disease, chronic obstructive pulmonary disease, diabetes, and cancer will be better characterized into many different sub-diseases rather than lumped into broad disease labels.

These subsets will be shown to have different genetic backgrounds with the potential to be responsive to treatment with oligomers that induce splice switching (or splice modulating) or translation suppressing.

Want a glimpse as to where the future could be headed? All you have to do is look at the oligomers that have already been approved and those that are in clinical studies in the U.S. right now.

Approved Oligomers

Currently fomivirsen (brand name Vitravene) is an antiviral drug that was developed by Isis Pharmaceuticals (see below) and is one of only two approved oligonucleotides. It was licensed by the U.S. Food and Drug Administration (FDA) in August 1998 and by the European Medicines Agency (EMA) in July 1999 for the treatment of cytomegalovirus retinitis (CMV) in patients with compromised immune systems, including those with AIDS. It was the first antisense antiviral, designed to inhibit the viral gene, approved by the FDA and was available by injection directly into the eyeball. It was marketed by the Swiss pharma giant, Novartis.

Fomivirsen blocks translation of viral mRNA by binding to a coding segment of a key CMV gene. Thus fomivirsen is an example of a Translation Suppressing Oligomer (TSO). Due to other advances in AIDS therapy and the dramatic decline in CMV retinitis, this drug is no longer marketed by Novartis.

Another novel approved oligonucleotide, pegaptanib, an aptamer (a single strand of DNA) is also injected directly into the eye. Pegaptanib works "downstream" by binding directly to a protein.

Oligomers in Clinical Development

Most clinical studies involving novel oligonucleotides can now be identified on ClinicalTrials.gov, or one of the other publically accessible registries. ClinicalTrials.gov currently has over 110,000 trials registered, with locations in over 170 countries. Of these trials, about 120 are listed as involving "oligonucleotides". Ten involve "oligomers".

The active or completed studies (as at July 2011) of therapeutic Antisense Oligonucleotides (AONs) or Oligomers [and their chemical name when determined] are listed in Table 7.1. It is only a "snapshot" as of July 2011 – to give an idea of how many companies, with how many oligomers, are currently being tested in humans with their drugs.

The oligomer that is farthest along is mipomersen. It has been developed for a subset of patients at risk of developing early severe coronary heart disease, CHD. Specifically, it has been designed for those genetically predisposed to very high levels of cholesterol. A new drug application for mipomersen, brand name Kynamro™, was submitted to the U.S. FDA in Spring 2012. In October 2012, mipomersen was reviewed by an FDA Advisory Committee who voted in favor of it being approved.

Oligomer (company name)	General disease area[1]	Sponsor company
EG35156	10 studies: Cancer	Aegera
ALN-RSV01	3 studies: RSV[2] infection	Alnylam
ALN-VSP02	2 studies: Cancer	
ALN-TTR02	Amyloidosis	
ARC1779	2 studies: Blood disorders	Archemix
AVI-4658 PMO[3] [Eteplirsen]	3 studies: Duchenne muscular dystrophy	AVI BioPharma
AVI-6002	1 study: Ebola virus hemorrhagic fever	
AVI-6003	1 study: Marburg virus hemorrhagic fever	
AVI-7100	1 study: Influenza	
L-Grb-2	Cancer	Biopath Holdings
EL625 [Cenersen]	2 studies: Cancer	Eleos
EZN-2968	2 studies: Cancer	Enzon
G3139 [Oblimersen]	45 studies: Cancer	Genta
IMO-2055	3 studies: Cancer	Idera
LEraf AON[4]	3 studies: Cancer	Insys
ISIS 3521	5 studies: Cancer	Isis
ISIS 5132	2 studies: Cancer	
ISIS 104838	Rheumatoid arthritis	
ISIS 2302 [Alicaforsen]	4 studies: Inflammatory bowel disease	
ISIS 113715	2 studies: Diabetes	
ISIS 301102 [Mipomersen]	13 studies: Hypercholesterolemia	
LOR-2040	2 studies: Crohn's disease	Lorus

NOX-E36	3 studies: Diabetes, Inflammatory disease	Noxxon
NOX-A12	2 studies: Blood disorders	
NOX-H94	Anemia	
OGX-427	3 studies: Cancer	OncoGenex
OGX-011 [Custirsen]	9 studies: Cancer	
PNT2258	Cancer	Pronai
PRO051	3 studies: Duchenne muscular dystrophy	Prosensa/GSK
PRO044	Duchenne muscular dystrophy	Prosensa
SPC5001	Hypercholesterolemia	Santaris
SPC4955	Hypercholesterolemia	
EMD1201081	Kidney cancer	Serono
ASM8-003	2 studies: Asthma	Topigen
c-mybASODN	Anemia	Univ of Penn

[1]Broad category of disease or specific disease. [2]RSV=Respiratory Syncytial Virus. [3]PMO=Phosphorodiamidate Morpholino Oligomer. A chemical class of oligomer based on a synthetic morpholino sugar, instead of the ribose and a phosphorodiamidate linkage instead of the more common phosphorothioate linkage. [4]AON=Antisense Oligonucleotide.

Table 7.1. The various oligomers in clinical development (July 2011).

Mipomersen Update

On January 29, 2013, Isis announced that the FDA had approved mipomersen. The first oligonucleotide for systemic administration can now be marketed. The time for oligonucleotides is nigh.

This drug will be a game changer. Coronary heart disease is responsible for one in four American deaths. It is the number one cause of death in the U.S. More than 400,000 Americans died from coronary heart disease in 2008. Every year, nearly 800,000 Americans have a first heart attack, and another 470,000 have a repeated heart attack. In 2012, coronary heart disease is expected to cost the U.S. over one hundred billion dollars for health care services, medicines and lost productivity.

Doctors are finding that there are multiple causes for coronary heart disease, only one of which is to have a genetic predisposition to high cholesterol. About 16% of Americans have high cholesterol. If you are one of those people, you have twice the risk of getting coronary heart disease as those who have normal levels of cholesterol.

The good news is that you are probably already getting tested for your cholesterol and you may know whether it is normal and how you can adjust your diet and increase your exercise to bring it down, if needed. If that doesn't work, one of a group of medicines called statins might be prescribed for you. Statins interfere with the biochemical pathway that generates cholesterol in your liver.

Lipitor, one of the statins manufactured by Pfizer is the top selling drug in the U.S., with another statin, Crestor, from Astra Zeneca at number eleven. These two statins generate total annual sales of nearly twenty billion dollars, and there are several others. However, the statins can also lead to side effects including muscle damage, so they don't suit everyone.

If you have high or very high levels of cholesterol you may have a genetic defect that creates high levels of lipids (fats) and their constituents in the blood stream, such as apoC-III, lipoprotein-A, low density lipoprotein (LDL)-C and triglyceride. These lipids are the cause of the high cholesterol you are experiencing. However, these other lipids are not targeted by the statins. The statin drug class only blocks synthesis of new cholesterol in the liver.

The good news is that the oligomers under development block the mRNA farther upstream, thereby reducing the production of apolipoprotein B. "ApoB" is found in the center of the devastating fatty plaques that build up inside blood vessels, including the coronary arteries, in the presence of high cholesterol, leading to their lethal blockage. Once a coronary artery is blocked you suffer from a heart attack.

There are approximately 40,000 patients in Europe and the U.S. who have inherited the condition above, known as Familial Hypercholesterolemia. If you are one of these, you have a genetic background that predisposes you to early, potentially fatal coronary heart disease. Unfortunately, you will not be able to lower your cholesterol levels by using a statin. But you may very well benefit from mipomersen, the new oligomer approved by the FDA in January of 2013.

Mipomersen was discovered and developed by the biopharmaceutical company, Isis, based in Carlsbad, California. (In 2008, Isis signed a deal with the Boston based biotech company, Genzyme, worth over one billion dollars. Genzyme was subsequently bought by the biggest French pharmaceutical company, Sanofi-Aventis.)

Mipomersen inhibits the generation of apolipoprotein (Apo) B-100. ApoB forms the core of the "bad" low density lipoprotein (LDL) cholesterol particles which float around in our bloodstream. Excessive LDL cholesterol forms the fatty plaques that build up on the inside of blood vessel walls in the heart. These fatty plaques grow to partially block the coronary arteries. Because the plaques also damage the blood vessel walls and form an irregular, inflamed surface, blood clots may form. This is the final straw and the already narrowed blood vessel becomes suddenly and completely blocked. This is what is meant by a heart attack.

Patients with an inherited condition called familial hypercholesterolemia have much higher levels of LDL-cholesterol, often unable to be controlled with strict low fat diet and maximum dose of the statin drugs. They are more likely to succumb to early coronary heart disease and fatal heart attacks. Mipomersen has been shown to reduce the elevated levels of LDL cholesterol by almost half compared to just diet and a statin, but no mipomersen.

Mipomersen is different from earlier oligonucleotides. It has an altered sugar backbone consisting of deoxyribose molecules, the same as in DNA, mixed with 2'-O-methoxyethyl-modified ribose. This mix of sugars makes the drug more resistant to breakdown by the body's enzymes, in this case nucleases. This greater stability and resistance to breakdown allows for mipomersen to be given by weekly administration, and makes it a so called "second generation" oligonucleotide. The drug accumulates in the liver, where it targets and blocks the mRNA that translates to the high levels of apoB.

Prior to its approval by the FDA, mipomersen completed four separate phase III trials (see Chapter 9) in patients with familial hypercholesterolemia (FH). All trials showed exceptional performance with the highest efficacy seen so far in both homozygous (hoFH - both chromosomes carry the FH gene) and heterozygous (heFH - only one of the two non-sex chromosomes carries the FH gene) populations. The oligomer was well tolerated, as suggested by the fact that few patients stopped their treatment. It is given by injection into the layers under the skin once weekly, with perhaps the biggest disadvantage being the pain of injection.

Other Oligomers in Development by Isis

Isis Pharmaceuticals, based in Carlsbad, California, has the broadest pipeline of any of the RNA-therapeutics companies, with numerous targets in different disease areas. Mipomersen is one of six oligomers they have developed. They have also been successful in seeking partnerships with several of the big pharmaceutical companies who will be able to support their oligomer development, as well as the commercialization of these products, which can be very expensive.

Typically, these partnerships have three phases. In the first phase, the larger company pays license fees to the innovator. In the second phase, both companies then share costs and responsibilities during clinical development often with milestone payments to the innovator as clinical steps are satisfactorily completed. Finally, in the third phase, the product is released commercially with the larger company providing marketing support and also sales representatives to promote the new drug to doctors in their offices. The original company receives royalties from the big pharma company. With these partnerships, Isis has generated more than $800 million since 2007 – funds that have been ploughed back into more early research.

Here's a list, by category, of the types of drugs Isis has in development as of July 2011, based on information on its website (www. isispharm.com/Pipeline/index.htm):

- Six cardiovascular drugs, one of which is in the last stage of development before approval
- Four drugs for severe and rare diseases, all in early stages of development
- Five drugs for metabolic illnesses in early stages of development
- Four drugs for treating cancer, including two in early development, one in a middle stage and one in an advanced stage that "inhibits the production of clusterin, a secreted protein that acts as a cell-survival protein and is overexpressed in response to cancer treatments, like chemotherapy, hormone ablation and radiation therapy."
- Seven drugs for inflammation and other miscellaneous ailments. One of these is in an early stage, four are in middle stages and two are in advanced stages, including both Vitravene, which

treats CMV retinitis in AIDS patients and Alicaforsen, used in the treatment of ulcerative colitis.

The lifeblood of innovative companies is to gain patent protection on their intellectual property and discoveries. That allows them to retain the "rights" to their ideas and either license out, or develop and market their drugs themselves, with protection from competition for the lifetime of the patent. Isis has designed and executed a patent strategy that has provided them with strong and extensive protection for their drugs as well as all aspects of oligomer discovery, development and manufacturing. Isis has over 1500 issued patents in their intellectual property portfolio and has earned more than $400 million from their intellectual property sale and licensing program as of July 2012.

Isis lists various attributes possessed by its antisense technology with the claim that these allow the building of a successful drug discovery platform and the creation of better drugs to benefit patients:

- **Specificity.** Oligomers are each designed to selectively target only one gene product. The more selectivity a drug has for its target, the better the drug.

- **Broad Applicability.** Complementary oligomers can be created for any RNA target, including targets that are considered "un-druggable" by traditional pharmaceuticals. Isis research is focused on diseases that are associated with RNA targets found in liver, kidney, spleen, bone marrow and fat cells where the oligomers tend to accumulate.

- **Rational Design.** Antisense oligomer discovery is more rational than any other type of drug discovery because:
  - o The rules for creating antisense drugs are known. They bind to target RNA.

o The monomer building blocks are constant for a particular chemistry. It is the order of these blocks (subunits) that directs the oligomer to a specific target.

o The distribution and metabolism of oligomers are very similar from drug to drug, with the same chemistry, leading to a common, predictable, safety profile.

- **Efficiency.** Developing new oligomers is much less costly and time consuming at the drug discovery and early development stages than traditional small molecule drugs. Lessons learned from the testing of one oligomer can lead to future oligomers, reducing the potential for early failures, resulting in significant competitive advantage for the platform.

- **Manufacturing.** Advances in process chemistry have resulted in dramatic reductions in the cost to manufacture these drugs.

Isis was founded by Dr. Stan Crooke and his colleagues in 1989. The Company completed its initial public offering in May 1991. Isis was the first company to commercialize an antisense drug (Vitravene) in 1998. In 2006, Dr. Crooke was named in Nature Biotechnology as one of biotechnology's influential individuals.

Oligomers in Development by Alnylam

Another pioneering company in nucleic acid-based therapeutics is Alnylam, based in Cambridge, Massachusetts, a biotechnology hub. Alnylam has focused its efforts on RNA interference, RNAi, to silence disease causing genes. Their oligomers are therefore Translation Suppressing Oligomers, as well as targeting microRNA which is yet another type of RNA whose structure and function is attracting increasing attention. Alnylam is named after the central star in the Orion constellation, which at 250,000 times brighter than the sun, represents to them the great potential that RNAi may have on human health. Alnylam recognizes that approximately eighty percent of the new targets that have been identified as a result of the Human Genome Project would be "un-druggable" with conventional drugs and biologics.

In 2004, Alnylam scientists demonstrated the ability to deliver oligomers to mice achieving a desired therapeutic effect. Then in 2006, Alnylam reported similar results in non-human primates; both of these landmark studies were published in the journal, Nature. In 2008, they showed that RNAi works in man when an oligomer, delivered locally, achieved statistically significant efficacy in a randomized, double-blind, placebo-controlled human clinical trial.

Alnylam expects to have five RNAi therapeutic products for genetically defined diseases in advanced stages of clinical development by the end of 2015. Alnylam has additional partner-based programs in clinical or development stages, including ALN-RSV01 for respiratory syncytial virus (RSV) infection, ALN-VSP for liver cancer, and ALN-HTT for Huntington's disease (Table 7.2 on next page).

As can be seen, Alnylam too has a rich pipeline of projects approaching, or already in, early clinical development. They are also taking aim at subsets of patients with coronary heart disease, anemia, and cancer.

Anemia is another diagnosis that hides many different pathologically distinct diseases. Until recently, the global prevalence of anemia was thought to be large but nobody knew the exact rate. Then in 1995-2005, the World Health Organization made a concerted effort to capture the data. In their report, they claim that approximately fifty percent of anemia is due to iron deficiency – which in turn is often related to inadequate iron intake, poor absorption (when the diet is high in certain iron binding compounds that prevent its absorption across

Drug	Target/Disease	Phase	Partner
ALN-TTR	Transthyretin I (TTR)/ Amyloidosis	I	Genzyme
ALN-TTR02[1]	TTR/ Amyloidosis	II	Genzyme
ALN-TTR$_{SC}$	TTR/ Amyloidosis	Preclinical	Genzyme
ALN-AT3	Antithrombin/ Hemophilia	Preclinical	Not yet
ALN-APC[2]	Protein C/ Hemophilia	Preclinical	Not yet
ALN-HPN[3]	Hepcidin/ Refractory anaemia	Preclinical	Not yet
ALN-TMP[4]	Transmembrane protease (serine 6)/ Anaemia, thalassemia and sickle cell disease	Preclinical	Not yet
ALN-PCS[5]	Proprotein convertase subtilisin/kexin (PCSK)9/ high cholesterol - CHD	I	Not yet
ALN-RSV01	Respiratory Syncytial Virus (RSV)	II	Cubist/ Kyowa Hakko Kirin
ALN-VSP	Kinesin spindle protein (KSP) and Vascular endothelial growth factor (VEGF)/ Cancer (liver)	I	Ascletis

OUT LICENSED PROGRAMS

Disease area	Oligomer	Phase	Partner
Diabetic macular edema	RTP801	II	Pfizer/Quark
Acute kidney injury	p53	I	Quark
Solid tumors	RRM2	I	Calando
Hypercholesterolemia	apoB	Development	Tekmira
Solid tumors	PLK1	Development	Tekmira
Hepatitis C	miR-122	Development	Regulus
JC Virus/PML		Discovery	BiogenIdec
Novartis programs	Various	Discovery	Novartis
Oncology & Metabolic	Various	Discovery	Takeda
Immuno-Inflammatory	Various (micro-RNA)	Discovery	GSK/Regulus
Heart failure/fibrosis	miR-21	Discovery	Regulus
Solid tumors	HIF-2α	Discovery	Calando
Solid tumors	DNA helicase	Discovery	GeneCare
Malaria	Various	Discovery	Cenix

[1][2][3][4][5] = *the five programs in Alnylam's 5 x15 strategy.*

Table 7.2. Alnylam's oligomer pipeline (as at July 16, 2012).

the gut wall), and periods in life when iron requirements may be higher. Such periods include childhood and pregnancy for women. Another cause of anemia is the heavy loss of iron through heavy menstruation or gastrointestinal parasites. Malaria in the tropics and almost any chronic illness can lead to hemoglobin levels dropping and the picture of iron deficiency. And a lack of certain other vitamins and minerals can lead to anemia, but not necessarily iron deficiency anemia.

The prevalence of anemia is different for various populations – both in terms of age within any given country and different between different regions of the globe. The WHO report, published in 2008, stated that anemia affects 1.6 billion people.

Sickle cell anemia has the clearest genetic components. As was discussed in chapter 4, sickle cell disease is caused by a single nucleotide change in the gene, an adenine base is changed for thymine. It has been proposed that oligonucleotides could be used combined with other agents to stop the production of the sickle cell mutant protein.

Although sickle cell disease, SCD, is primarily a disease of Africans, the ebb and flow of populations around the world means that it is common in the U.S. as well, with an estimated one hundred thousand Americans affected. Over a four-year period from 1989 to 1993, SCD was blamed for 75,000 hospitalizations in the U.S. costing us $475 million in healthcare. Thus an effective treatment for SCD would have both a U.S. and global benefit.

Another genetic cause of iron deficiency anemia is thalassemia. Thalassemia is caused by either a deletion or mutation of the globin regulatory genes leading to a reduced number of normal globin molecules. Like SCD, thalassemia carrier status (those with only one affected gene, not two) appears to offer a survival advantage against malaria. Up to 18% of the population in the island nation of the Maldives and 16% of the population of Cypress are carriers of an affected gene.

Currently the only treatment for thalassemia, in severe cases, is a blood transfusion with normal red blood cells.

More than ten years ago, Professor Ryszard Kole and his colleagues took cells from patients with beta thalassemia and treated them with a Splice Switching Oligomer. This led to a seventy percent increase in correctly spliced beta globin mRNA and a subsequent 36% increase in hemoglobin. Kole's experiment was one of the earliest examples of Splice Switching, although in this case it was done in cells after their removal from the patient.

Sadly, although 181 clinical studies are registered for the treatment of thalassemia there are currently no studies exploring the benefits of oligomers. It's time for companies to realize that sickle cell disease and thalassemia could be amenable to this kind of treatment. Hopefully the Alnylam program (ALN-TMP) will soon advance into the clinic with their anti-thalassemia oligomer.

Oligomers presently represent only a fraction of the novel drugs being reviewed at the FDA. There are approximately two hundred new drugs being taken into the early stages of human testing each year by industry. At the moment, only about 15 oligomers per year enter human testing. This imbalance will lessen as the number of novel small molecule drugs edging into the clinic continues to decline, while the number of oligomers increases, especially now that mipomersen is approved.

Oligomers in Development by Other Companies

Many other companies have a plethora of DNA-defying drugs in the pipeline. Here's a snapshot of which companies are testing oligomers in human studies and what diseases they're working on:

- Antisense Pharma, from the German biotechnology center of Regensburg, with advanced programs with trabedersen for ten different cancers, including phase II studies in pancreatic cancer, glioma (a brain cancer) and malignant melanoma (a skin cancer)

- Silence Therapeutics of London, UK, is working with short interfering RNA (siRNA) oligomers in acute kidney injury, cancer and lung disease. Silence has partnerships with Astra-Zeneca, Pfizer, Novartis, Quark Pharma, Novartis, and Dainippon Sumitomo.

- Santaris Pharma of Horsholm, Denmark with clinical programs in hepatitis C (with miravirsen), cancer (solid tumors), and hypercholesterolemia. They too have formed partnerships for their less advanced programs with some of the bigger pharmaceutical companies - Shire, Pfizer and GlaxoSmithKline.

- Quark Pharmaceuticals with labs in Fremont, California, as well as Boulder, Colorado and Israel, has programs with Pfizer in diabetic eye disease and with Novartis in acute kidney injury and after kidney transplantation.

- Regado Biosciences of Basking Ridge, New Jersey and Durham, North Carolina has a technology that uses a two-component system to help prevent blood clots. Regado uses aptamers (usually small strands of DNA or RNA, but can also be of peptide and can occur naturally) that bind to clotting factors, preventing clots from forming, followed by an oligomer that binds to and neutralizes the aptamer.

- Topigen based in Montreal, Canada is now part of the Sydney, Australia-based Pharmaxis. Topigen has been developing ASM8, an inhaled combination of two oligomers for severe allergic asthma. They announced successful results from a phase II clinical study in April 2012, and represent the exciting possibility that inhaled oligomers may successfully target lung disease.

- Prosensa, a Dutch company, has two programs in Duchenne muscular dystrophy patients, each targeting a different Exon, 51 and 44. They are partnered with GlaxoSmithKline.
- Sarepta Therapeutics, my former employer, has programs in DMD, too. Their most advanced is also aimed at Exon 51, with earlier programs targeting other exons. They are also testing oligomers against Ebola and Marburg hemorrhagic fevers and influenza. The latter has just been partnered with a branch of the U.S. National Institutes of Health.

As can be seen there are several companies looking at the application of oligomer therapies for various cancers. This represents a challenge but also an opportunity. Many different types of cancer are due to genetic mutations that often are passed down from your parents. Sometimes however a new mutation may occur in our children. The most well-known cancer-associated genes are BRCA1 and BRCA2, which predispose for a greater risk of cancer of the breast for both genders, and for the ovary in women. These genes are now so well recognized that a woman with one of these genes may be offered a prophylactic mastectomy where her breasts could be removed in an attempt to thwart her genetic destiny.

Several other cancers are now known to be associated with certain gene mutations, including cancers of the colon, rectum, thyroid gland, and prostate. An association, however, is not a cause. Cancer is a complex disease and not only must your genes put you at increased risk, but you need to be exposed to one or more environmental triggers that will also be involved in turning on the cancer cells. Some cancer-associated genes regulate the production of cancer growth stimulators, while others switch off the production of healthy chemicals that get rid of early cancer cells. As these cancer-promoting genes and their products have become better understood, there has been a surge of interest in developing oligomers to block their effect by translation suppression.

More recently, however, splice switching oligomers have been considered for cancer therapy. One experiment has even shown that the redirection of splicing was effective at reducing the spread of malignant melanoma cells in skin cancer.

Frustratingly, in March 2012, scientists from the UK's Cancer Research Institute noted that even within the same kidney cancer, different mutations of a gene were found. Additionally, when the cancer spread to other organs, different genes were switched on. It's far from clear how doctors will incorporate this new information into decisions about which current small molecule or new oligomeric drugs to offer any individual patient.

This research helped explain why existing medicines against cancer in patients have not been as effective as predicted from test tube or animal experiments.

Relatively few companies are working on developing oligomers however for other common diseases at this time. Why is that?

Since "antisense" was first discussed in the literature in the 1980s, it has been estimated that over ten billion dollars in total has been spent on research and development, with only two drugs, fomivirsen and pegaptanib, gaining approval. Neither has been a commercial success.

Isis, Alnylam, and Sarepta Therapeutics started on their development programs in the 80s and 90s. Then several first generation oligomers failed in their clinical testing programs. The prevailing enthusiasm dissipated and an article even appeared in *Nature* in 1995 with the title "Does Antisense Exist?"

In the new millennium, interest recovered with the discovery of a different mechanism of action for the RNA targeting oligomers, that of RNA interference by Fire and Mello (see below) which was described as the breakthrough of the year in 2002. With another ten years of effort, RNA targeting oligomers have now been developed that operate in twelve distinct ways, and there are over fifty oligomers in development. To make the scientific and regulatory challenges greater, these various oligomers also have a variety of different chemistry backbones. That makes the task of achieving consistent results challenging. It also makes it harder to attract bigger companies to invest in the small companies doing the research. Those large companies, and their massive bank accounts, are often necessary to take the new drugs into an expensive clinical program, which can now cost ten to one hundred million dollars.

Big Pharma

The biggest pharmaceutical companies are letting smaller companies take the initial steps in developing oligomers. They are waiting for the latest nucleic acid-based therapeutics to get to a later stage of development before they get involved. Once the oligomers are approved, they'll lend their marketing muscle to the innovating company. But they'll do so without having had to acquire the oligomer, or the innovator company, and take on all the risks in the process. Nonetheless, they'll still make a sizable profit if one of these drugs becomes a hit.

America's Pfizer, the largest pharmaceutical company, is working on development projects with Alnylam and Quark. The Swiss company, Novartis, also has license deals with Alnylam, although they seem less enthusiastic now, having passed on the option to license Alnylam's RNAi intellectual property. The British pharmaceutical giant, GSK, is working with Prosensa on their lead PRO051 phosphorothioate oligomer in DMD and has options on their other oligomers in development. Merck acquired the San Francisco based siRNA Therapeutics in December of 2006, whose technology involves activating the RNA-Induced Silencing Complex (RISC), but has not yet entered clinical trials. Nevertheless, siRNA has demonstrated efficacy in animal models of disease and is now known to be abundant in eukaryotic cells where they exert control over how much mRNA is expressed. So the large companies are hedging their bets with regard to oligomers.

RNA interference, RNAi, was first reported in an article by Andrew Fire and Craig Mello in Nature in 1998. They showed that small snippets of double stranded RNA, dsRNA, could shut down genes and prevent the translation of mRNA into protein. Their attempt was much better than the previous ones with single stranded RNA. In 2001, the process was demonstrated in mammalian cells. The next year Alnylam was founded and in 2004 RNAi was shown to work in an experiment on a live animal. Fire and Mello were awarded the Nobel Prize in Medicine in 2006 *"for their discovery of RNA interference - gene silencing by double-stranded RNA"* which has opened up a whole new field in biology.

By 2010, thirty scientists had been awarded Nobel Prizes for experimental work on RNA – a testament to the molecule's importance to life on earth.

The problem with oligomers, as with stem cells and gene therapy, is that they all tend to work in the laboratory when dripped onto cell culture in experiments. But it is much harder to get them to enter and work on the appropriate cells in whole live animals, let alone in humans.

Some of these issues have now been overcome in the last few years and many more oligomers are now in clinical development. Several of them are using sophisticated chemical modification to make them more stable and resistant to the body's attempt to destroy them, as well as to help them enter cells and penetrate into the nucleus.

Summary

For now, smaller entrepreneurial biotech and biopharmaceutical companies are tasked with the research and development of RNA modulating oligomers. The path to approval remains long, expensive and in some cases unclear. Many of the diseases currently being targeted by oligomers have previously been considered "un-druggable" and hence experience with conducting clinical studies in these lethal, inexorable childhood diseases is limited. How successful the new oligomers will be depends on many things, not least the various chemical modifications made.

Setbacks have been overcome in previous new medicine classes. The early monoclonal antibody programs of the eighties had repeated failures and setbacks, yet only three decades later, four of the top ten drugs by revenue are monoclonal antibodies, each generating in excess of six billion dollars. The recent economic downturn has surely slowed the progress of some of the oligomers in development, and postponed plans for others. Recently, more than one hundred thousand employees were laid off by pharmaceutical companies in the U.S. alone, but the diseases will not go away. Once market conditions improve and investors feel encouraged by the promise of nucleic acid-based therapeutics, the race will heat up again. Will all the oligomers discussed above make it to market? Possibly not. But as with the monoclonal antibodies, enough oligomers may make it over all the regulatory hurdles for a new era of highly targeted, RNA-sequence specific, personalized medicines, to become a reality.

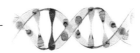

Chapter Eight

The Doctor's Office
of the Future

octors face an onslaught of new genetic discoveries that promise to fundamentally alter the way they learn, practice, view, and prescribe medicine. The idealistic image of your caring physician attending you when you are sick is transforming into a new picture: doctors as learned partners who, armed with genetic knowledge about you, can help you prevent illness in the first place.

In this fast changing world, if you have a genetic predisposition for a disease or a single disease-causing gene, who will be your advocate? Who will have the time, knowledge, and ability to explain the science behind these new oligomer therapies and whether you may need one? There will still be a role for the doctor as scientist and compassionate, proactive healer in this new paradigm.

Currently if you are at risk of, or have, a genetically determined disease the doctor you are most likely to consult with is the local clinical geneticist. Your local genetics clinic will have trained counselors as well as physicians skilled in interpreting the mass of genetic information potentially available to you today. These teams are now routinely brought in when new babies appear to be abnormal, or when there is a strong family history of a disease. They are frequently also consulted by pregnant women who may be at risk of bearing a baby with genetic problems.*

Also, they are helpful to some oncologists who make cancer treatment decisions based on genetic information. The range of medical and surgical sub-specialties where genetics makes an impact continues to grow, so clinical geneticists will grow busier and busier every year.

In the future, all doctors will need to be prepared to deal with basic genetics questions. And your doctor's role will continue to evolve as more genetic diseases are identified. With the new wave of oligomers, many genetic ailments will be treatable. These illnesses will require accurate, early diagnosis and patients will still need sympathetic counseling. This will especially be true while the wheels of drug development turn at a pace that frustrates and confounds society.

Some companies are already offering insight into your genome. Many doctors are uneasy about direct to consumer genetic testing as it may stir up unnecessary anxiety, even with good counseling support. In addition the testing may occasionally identify unexpected paternity and bring families into crisis. However, in the absence of regulation, we have such testing available now from several companies.

23andME, based in Mountain View, California, was founded in 2006 and began offering DNA testing in 2007. Its founders include the wife of one of Google's founders. In 2008, the 23andME (so named

---

* Historically, testing for a possible Down's syndrome baby (or other chromosomal abnormality) has been offered to women by a test called amniocentesis. In early pregnancy, fluid is taken from the amniotic cavity surrounding the growing baby. Some of the baby's cells will be floating in this fluid. However, we now recognize that some of the baby's DNA can be found floating freely in the mother's bloodstream from early in pregnancy, so amniocentesis will eventually be replaced by a blood test.

for the 23 pairs of human chromosomes) personal genome testing kit, which requires a spit sample only, was named "Invention of the Year" by Time magazine. Currently the spit sample lets 23andME look at 960,000 single nucleotide polymorphisms or SNPs.

That is not the whole genome, but ultimately, sequencing the whole genome is their goal.

The SNPs assess risk for 119 inherited diseases and provides information about your ancestry. The test allows predictions to be made about how you will respond to certain frequently prescribed drugs.

Initially, the states of California and New York tried to block 23andMe from offering their services to their residents, but they were unsuccessful. The company is currently licensed to provide services in California. Now, for $299, you can request the spit sample kit, send it in and get information on your risk of contracting one or more of the following diseases:

- Alzheimer's disease
- Asthma
- Bipolar disorder
- Bladder, breast, lung or prostate cancer
- Chronic lymphocytic leukemia
- Coronary heart disease
- Cystic fibrosis
- Diabetes
- Lou Gehrig's disease (ALS)
- Multiple sclerosis
- Obesity
- Schizophrenia
- Sickle Cell anemia

This list is just a small sample of common diseases, but there are many rare diseases covered by the 23andMe test.

The test will also provide information on 48 carrier states, also known as disease traits.

A carrier state means that you have one of the recessive genes and can pass the disease to 1 in 4 of your children if you mate with another carrier.

Having a disease trait means the same thing—that you only have one of the two recessive genes that are required to give you the disease. If you actually have a disease, you will either have both of the pair of recessive genes or one dominant gene.

Navigenics offers sequencing direct to the public. They were founded in 2006 in Foster City, California. In 2012, Navigenics was acquired by Life Technologies, a large instrument, reagent, and technical services supplier based in Carlsbad, California. Life Technologies formed in 2008 with the merger of two successful but smaller equipment and reagent manufacturers: Invitrogen and Applied Biosystems. Their equipment is some of the most advanced and robust for analyzing genetic information and sequencing your genome. In July 2012, their machine, the Ion Proton entered the Genomic X Prize to sequence the full human genome for under one thousand dollars, and within one day.

A third company in this market, one that I actually received a report from, is deCODEme genetics. Founded in 1996 in Reykjavik, Iceland with the aim of identifying genes associated with common diseases on the basis of population studies, deCODEme successfully identified genes associated with heart disease, cancer and schizophrenia.

The company launched its web-based personal genome service in November 2007. For a fee of $985 and a swab from inside your cheek, they look for evidence of 47 diseases. They accomplish this task by scanning more than one million SNPs. The range of disease they look at is similar to the range from 23andMe.

In 2006, deCODE launched a lawsuit against five former employees who, they allege, took trade secrets with them and joined the Children's Hospital of Philadelphia. deCODEme filed for bankruptcy in 2009. Their assets were bought by an investment company in 2010 who have continued to support most of their services. In December 2012, California-based biotherapeutics company Amgen bought deCODE for $415 million.

In 2012, I was able to go online and obtain a demonstration of what their report would look like – for one genetic disease I am at risk for – heart disease (Figure 8.1).

I have slightly under the average risk of suffering a heart attack, according to my genetics, as a male of European ancestry. Now it is up to me to take that report to my doctor and discuss how I might reduce that risk by altering my environment and my behavior. There is nothing I can do to alter my genes.

Sequencing your whole genome for under one thousand dollars and in less than 24 hours will be here soon. Some companies will work directly with consumers. Others will only allow doctors to request their reports. Although the consumer companies will offer advice based on your results, your doctor will be the best person to help you interpret the mass of information and advice you are likely to get. He or she will help you decide which bits of advice are realistic for you and which may need to be postponed.

In addition, by the end of this decade, some of the genetic messages giving rise to disease may have "gene-patch" medicines approved to combat them.

The new medicines will only be given to you by prescription and because many of them will be developed for rare disease, with limited stocks held in warehouses, distributing the drug to you will become highly sophisticated. Many of the gene patches will only be given by highly trained doctors specializing in your disease, and able to carefully monitor the effects of the drug. But your personal physician will, as always, be there for back up, to monitor your general health and care for you if any emergency arises. Thus he or she will need to understand your new treatment; how it is helping and what side effects to look out for, if any.

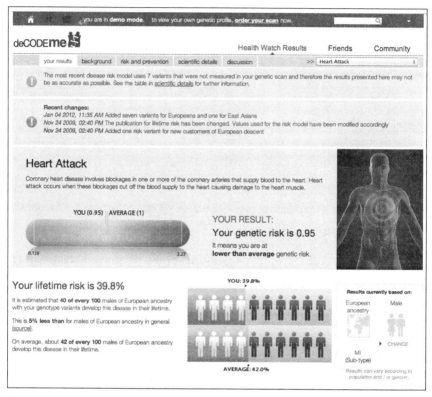

Figure 8.1. Demonstration report from deCODEme for my risk of suffering a heart attack.

Consultations of the Future

As the new era of medicine unfolds and genome sequencing becomes cheaper, quicker and more accessible, consultations with doctors will have a different tenor. Here are two conversations I imagine taking place in a world where we can defy our DNA. The first is with Mrs.

Singh, the mother of Deepak, the little boy with Duchenne muscular dystrophy from the beginning of this book.

In this scenario, imagine that I was able to take a routine sample from Deepak at birth – perhaps a small piece of the placenta, or some blood from the now severed umbilical cord. Mrs. Singh is now coming back for her routine checkup at six weeks after delivery. She is bringing baby Deepak for his first review.

I ask how things are going with him.

Mrs. Singh: "Deepak is feeding and sleeping well."

Me: "I am glad to hear that, Mrs. Singh.

We have the routine tests back from the samples we took when Deepak was born. We get a laboratory to analyze the samples to see if Deepak has any faulty genes that may cause illness now, or as he grows up.

"I am afraid that there is one gene that appears to be faulty. The faulty gene will cause him to have trouble with his muscles as he grows up. He has a disease called Duchenne muscular dystrophy. The good news is that over the last few years, we have developed a new type of treatment for this rare disease. Now for many boys, and Deepak is one of those, we can stop the faulty gene from causing the disease. With this new gene patch medicine, we can help Deepak grow up normally, with working muscles and lead a normal, healthy, active, happy life."

Mrs. Singh: "Oh Doctor. I am sad to hear Deepak will become ill. When will the illness start? Will the gene patch cure him?"

Me: "Usually boys start to have trouble after age three when they may start to stumble. In the past, the disease would be a slow killer, nearly always leading to their death before their thirtieth birthday.

By then they would be completely paralyzed. But with the new gene patch, Deepak will be fine. It won't cure him, but it will help him to make a replacement protein for one that is missing in his muscles now.

"He will need to take the treatment for the rest of his life, starting as soon as possible so that he develops normally. The medicine will be given as an injection, every week for a few weeks, then every month, and as he gets older, probably only once every two to three months. But he will need careful watching throughout his development."

Mrs. Singh: "How safe are these new genes?"

Me: "Well, this new treatment is not a new gene. Deepak will still have all of the genes he was born with. We are not replacing any of them. Maybe one day we will be able to replace the faulty gene with a healthy gene, but not yet. The faulty gene makes a faulty message – and in Deepak's case a vital protein, called dystrophin, is not made. The gene patch medicines act like a sort of Band-Aid on this faulty molecular message, repairing it so that his muscle cells make a replacement protein.

"As far as we can tell now, these gene patch treatments are well tolerated. But they are fairly new and nobody has taken them for very long yet, let alone a lifetime. That is why we will need to keep a close watch on Deepak as he grows."

Mrs. Singh: "What will happen if Deepak doesn't get this new treatment? What are the other options?"

Me: "Well, he will probably appear to be normal for a few years. But when he is three, or maybe five, you will notice he has difficulty walking, or running, or getting up from the floor. By the time he is ten, he won't be able to walk as his leg muscles will be too weak. Some boys do well with leg braces, but even they end up needing a wheelchair. Then in his teens his arms will get weaker and his breathing muscles will stop working well. He will need artificial breathing support. By the time he reaches age twenty, his heart muscle will also be affected.

"I should also warn you that the dystrophin protein that is missing in the muscles is also missing in the brain and many of the Duchenne boys have mental problems.

"There are no other effective treatments for Duchenne muscular dystrophy. For many years, affected boys have been treated with steroids that seem to slow some of the muscle loss – but only for a year or two. The steroids themselves cause many side effects over time which complicate boys' care. Until recently, the boys could end up also having many operations on their legs and back, as well as spending increasing amounts of time in the hospital. You may need to adapt your home to make it easier for wheelchair access. There are several organizations that can provide you with help and advice and put you in contact with other parents who have had to face the same situation. With the new medicine, Deepak should remain active and won't need steroids, leg braces, wheelchair, breathing support or, hopefully, any other medicines."

Mrs. Singh: "Why us? What did I do wrong in my pregnancy?"

Me: "You did nothing wrong! We are none of us perfect. Our genes sometimes develop faults when they are passed to our children. Sometimes this disease can run in families – and women can "carry" the affected gene but not get the disease. We should take a sample from you to check for that – but not today. Many of these cases of muscular dystrophy cannot be predicted or prevented – at least not yet. Maybe one day.

Mrs. Singh: "Can I bring my husband with me to talk to you?"

Me: "Of course. I would like to give you some leaflets, websites, and phone numbers for some of the Duchenne charities as well as the Muscular Dystrophy Association. I would encourage you to call them and talk to them. Perhaps they can put you in touch with other local parents you can meet. Then, when you and your husband want to come and talk to me about Deepak's diagnosis and the treatment, we can make time for you."

With that the first of many consultations would come to an end. I used to be sad and exhausted after telling a family of a new baby that he had such a terrible disease. Now, however the future is looking brighter for many with the rare Duchenne muscular dystrophy.

*****

Only one in every ten Americans has a rare disease. What would a doctor's appointment look like for the other nine Americans in a post-gene patch world?

John Smith, is a slightly overweight forty-five year old sales representative for a Silicon Valley semiconductor company. He stopped smoking over ten years ago and claims to have put on more weight since. He had his genome sequenced recently by a commercial, "direct to consumer" laboratory and called to ask if he could come and discuss the results with me.

John: "Good morning, Doc. I wanted to get your take on my genes after I got them checked out recently. Here are the results."

He thrusts a sheet of paper at me with a red circle around a figure of 1.68. This is his genetic risk of suffering a heart attack. It is nearly double the average risk.

Me: "Thank you. Firstly – you should be congratulated that you stopped smoking when you did. Your risk of a heart attack would be much higher if you hadn't. However, there is no room for complacency. This indicates that, based on just your genetics, you have a much greater than average chance of having a heart attack.

"Now we should look at your weight, cholesterol, and blood pressure as well as other tests for your heart. With those results, in addition to your genetic risk, we can build a more complete picture.

"There is nothing you can do about your genes, John, but you can reduce some of the other risk factors like you did when you stopped smoking. I am talking about taking regular, vigorous exercise, losing twenty to thirty pounds so you are at your ideal weight, and reducing your cholesterol. Your bad cholesterol has been just above the upper level of what is acceptable for the last few years. You did not want to take any treatment for it before, but given your increased genetic risk, you need to try and reduce this more seriously now. I can give you some suggestions about your diet, or I could arrange for you to see our nutritionist. If it doesn't come down with a better diet and more exercise, you should reconsider starting some cholesterol lowering treatment.

"Your blood pressure has always been pretty good, so I am not worried about that. We should check it today however. And as you are now in your mid-forties we should get an electrical recording of your heart. If you had had any bouts of chest pain – perhaps going upstairs or with exercise, I would want to look at the state of the blood vessels supplying your heart in more detail.

"By checking out these risk factors we can get a far more complete picture of your overall risk of getting a heart attack. Although your genes do contribute to that risk, they are only one of the many pieces in the overall picture. I would recommend that you start taking a low dose of aspirin every day. That has good evidence for reducing the risk of heart attack.

"Is there anything else that you are worried about?"

John: "Well doc, what about drinking? Can I still drink beer? And what about these new gene patch medicines that everyone is talking about these days?"

Me: "Alcohol in moderation has been shown to be beneficial and to actually lower the risk of heart disease. It still adds to calories, so you should balance your total calorie intake. You should also of course not drink and drive. You would lose your job if you lost your license – so be careful where and when you drink. Some people think red wine is more protective for your heart – and I believe that – but others say two to three units of alcohol per day for men helps, irrespective of what sort of alcohol it is.

"The new gene patch therapies – we call them oligomers – can be very useful for some very specific situations. The test you had did not specifically look for the genetic causes of high cholesterol. But if you had the rare genetic high cholesterol, your levels would have been much higher and we would have had to do something about them a long time ago. So I think it is most unlikely that you will need any of the new gene patch drugs. In time there may be more of them, treating a wider range of diseases, so we should keep an eye on developments."

Sometime in the near future, companies may be required to identify at-risk patients much more carefully during clinical development. Once approved, the label (and promotion) will encourage the new drug to be given only to those patients carefully selected on the basis of their genome. To get that drug, you may need to have your genes tested to see if you are suitable for it and for your insurer to pay for it.

Doctors will be the gatekeepers for these drugs, keeping your personal gene chart in their files so they can check them before they prescribe any medicine. If a medicine could cause heart problems in less than .001% of the population (one chance in one hundred thousand), but affects people with a particular gene, one that you have, then your physician will know to prescribe something else for you. Indeed, one day your genetic information will be programmed onto your doctor's medical records database and a warning will flash up if he tries to prescribe a drug to you that may cause problems. In fact, pretty soon we should be able to take our medical records, including our genetic information, with us everywhere. It could be put on a credit card or on a small storage device on our wrist or round our neck. If you are unlucky enough to be involved in an accident, paramedics will be able to read these details and ensure you get the right drugs while still at the scene. In addition, the rescue services can transmit the information to the ER at the local hospital so that they can be prepared and have your exact blood type ready for you in case it's needed.

Your genetic background could conceivably be used for multiple purposes. This may be the most exciting use of personalized medicine of all.

One day, common diseases like schizophrenia will be accurately diagnosed based on your specific genome sequence. That would allow the exact genetic mutation predisposing you to a certain pattern of schizophrenic illness to be clarified. In addition, your ability to metabolize drugs can be predicted and which dose of what drug will be best, and for how long it will be required. Or an alternative treatment could be precisely aimed at the RNA message within the cell, way upstream in the disease process from where schizophrenia and many other common diseases are being treated today.

In parallel, one or more biological measures (called biomarkers), like those found in a CAT scan or a blood panel, will be developed that detect the early warnings of untreated or inadequately treated schizophrenia. Thus a debilitating psychiatric disease, poorly treated by many of today's therapeutic options may be predicted on the basis of your genome, prevented by the administration of a specific oligomer, its effect monitored, and benefit confirmed by one or more biomarker.

Training Doctors in the Age of Personalized Medicine

As the role of physician continues to evolve, intrinsic changes must occur in training, office practice, and access to care.

Doctors involved in clinical research appreciate that genetics will need to be built into future clinical studies. Currently, blood samples are taken and stored under strict security from subjects in many studies, to test later. This is to permit genetic questions to be asked if a small proportion of subjects in a study do very well, or very badly. Do they share a good gene, or a bad one?

In the future, a huge, secure database will be available before a drug study even starts. Specially trained doctors will be able to go into that database and ask confidential questions about the disease they want to study; about what sort of people have that disease and what medicines they are currently taking. People will not be identifiable in this database, but it will be linked with other databases, so that your doctor can be alerted to a new drug being tested that may be ideal for you. Then, when you next visit your doctor, or ring in for a new prescription, or get called to go for a checkup, the new drug study might be something for you to discuss with your doctor.

As a new drug is tested, doctors will be able to ask this database what gene or genes may make subjects respond favorably or adversely to the new drug being tested. If the drug is similar to one already developed, that question may be easy to answer from information already gathered. Then those subjects with a "good" gene can be sought specifically and enrolled. Those with a "bad" gene can be excluded from the drug study.

Thus, genetics and genotyping will become common in every study and clinical research doctors will need to understand how it is done and what the implications of any results are. They will need to explain the findings to subjects who are interested in participating in the research and be able to answer any questions that subjects may have. In the case of oligomers being developed for genetic diseases, testing will only take place on those patients who have been confirmed to have a highly specific genetic makeup.

If your doctor does clinical research, then he or she is already used to the accelerating pace of change and increasing complexity of the regulations governing research.

Typical office practices will change in many other ways in this new genomic age.

Protecting your privacy and treating your medical records as confidential is well ingrained in medical care. But with the unraveling of the Human Genome, more questions crop up. For instance, what information should be provided to insurance companies? And how will they deal with genetic information that may be provided to you months if not years before a disease manifests?

Computerization of records and the potential for vast amounts of information to be instantly available on the other side of the world has so far not made medical records as transportable as they could be. That will come in time. Perhaps when you move to a new area with new doctors, you will be able to take an electronic copy of all your previous records. That could potentially be very helpful as previous illness, investigations, drug treatment and your response to it, with accurate dates, are quickly integrated with your new doctor's records of your consultation today.

Not all doctors do clinical research. But all doctors will be affected by genome sequencing. Without the need for a blood sample, whole families, including children, will be signing up to learn their genetic destiny. Health insurance companies will have worked out whether they will reimburse for these tests and what to do with the results. As more experience is gained with the interpretation of the results, your doctor will be the one to suggest specific treatment for you.

Over the next decade, development of therapeutic oligomers will gather momentum and there will be gene patches for many more ailments. As more diseases are identified before they cause you symptoms, your doctor will be able to offer you tools to prevent them from ever erupting. This will truly herald a Golden Age of Medicine.

As this occurs, upholding the Hippocratic Oath and the concept of "first do no harm" will be just as important as it is today. Doctors will need to understand not just the principles of genome sequencing, but also the seriousness of your identified condition and the timeline for your disease to manifest. They will then guide you through the mass of often competing claims about what environmental factors you can control and how your behavior may contribute to accelerating the disease, or conversely protecting you against it. Ultimately your doctor will be the one to confirm that you should receive one of the new gene patch medicines and then monitor your progress on it.

It is indeed a joy, and a privilege, to provide comfort, hope and the prescription of an effective medicine. Knowing that the drug being prescribed will make a difference in someone's life is the most rewarding part of the job of being a physician. I wish I could have prescribed an effective, life-saving drug for Deepak all those years ago. But my son and his generation of doctors will be able to prescribe effective oligomers for many boys with Duchenne muscular dystrophy and other rare disorders.

Many physicians have become adept at talking to patients and empowering families to take more control of their own health.

Sequencing your genome will make a diagnosis definitive. There has been nothing so clear and unequivocal before. Therefore, to give definitive answers to patients, doctors will start using the power of sequencing more and more often and earlier in life. Your genes do not change as you get older, so once your genome sequence is obtained, it will never need to be repeated.

All physicians are now required to undergo continuing medical education, which most conscientiously pursue anyway. This process allows them to stay up to date with diagnosis and/or treatment guidelines. In the next decade, genome sequencing and the many options available for patients will enter ongoing education for your physician, whatever branch or subspecialty of medicine they practice. Medicine is a rapidly changing science, and to be professionally competent requires ongoing education until retirement.

Your doctor will retain his or her role of providing you with the diagnoses, referring to specialists, counseling you and your family, and arranging for you to receive the appropriate treatment and care. Your doctor will continue to supervise administration of your therapy and monitor your progress sometimes for months, or years, or even for the remainder of your life. If you move, or your doctor retires, your electronic medical records will be available instantly to a new doctor.

Personal genomics will greatly reduce the chance for errors, especially of diagnosis, but errors of advice and interpretation will still remain. Doctors should receive support and encouragement to keep up to date and rectify any knowledge gaps or behavioral inadequacies, so that they can continue practicing the highest quality of care in this rapidly changing world. I hope that the Golden Age of Medicine will also be an enlightened age where medical mistakes and malpractice lawsuits become even rarer than the diseases that are untreatable today.

Summary

The arrival of the Human Genome Project and subsequent sequencing of the human genome has helped to diagnose more genetic diseases earlier. It has added impetus to the development of oligomers for rare, previously untreatable conditions. Further advances in genome sequencing herald more changes to the way medicine can benefit society to come. Sequencing the whole genome has helped define the single gene mutations for 2,900 rare diseases. It is only a matter of time before the genetic mutation that causes a further 3,600 other rare diseases are discovered. Sequencing the whole genome is predicted to drop below one thousand dollars in the near future.

In addition, it is thought that there may be another 4,500 disorders that have not yet been fully clinically characterized that may be attributable to single gene mutations. And there are at least 14,000 rare genetic diseases in all. Once all these have been described and those suitable for splice switching or translation suppressing by oligomers have been identified, the race will be on to develop oligomers for these conditions. Once developed, doctors will need to remain vigilant to the potential diagnoses, counseling made available to you and your family and explanations about the prognosis even as the drugs are going through the development process. Your physician will then be expected to choose the right oligomer for the right condition at the right dose, administer it at the right time and monitor your response with the right tools at the right frequency. With so many newly diagnosable diseases and so many novel oligomers being developed, the doctors of the future will have to face a lot more training both initially, and as continuing education. But the results will be worth it.

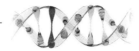

Chapter Nine

How Are New Drugs Regulated?

The biotechnology and pharmaceutical industries are the most highly regulated global industry. Why is this so? Formal regulation was needed to stop inappropriate labeling and extravagant claims about medicines that were downright lies.

Drug development regulation is overseen by the three main agencies, the Food and Drug Administration (FDA) in the U.S., the European Medicines Agency (EMA) in Europe and the Pharmaceuticals and Medical Devices Agency (PMDA) in Japan. Regulation of drug development started relatively recently.

Some argue that the regulations have become too burdensome, but a glaring example of the disaster that can happen when there is insufficient regulatory oversight is the outbreak of meningitis in October 2012.

A compounding pharmacy in Massachusetts made up steroid injections without seemingly obeying the usual sterility rules. The basic ingredient was contaminated with a fungus that was neither detected nor eliminated in the process of filling the vials for distribution. By the end of November 2012, 541 cases of meningitis had been confirmed in patients who had received a steroid injection into their spine. Fluid circulates in the meningeal space up and down the spine and around the brain, and the fungus was introduced into this fluid during the procedure. By the time the outbreak was recognized, the contaminated vials had already been distributed to 19 states. By early December 2012, the Center for Disease Control in Atlanta, Georgia, reported that 36 patients had already died.

The FDA was not given the close cooperation to contain, investigate and recall the faulty material that the pharmaceutical industry would have been expected to provide. Attorneys are lining up to sue the hapless manufacturer, the New England Compounding Center, and both civil and criminal charges are likely. This incident will prompt a review and tightening of the rules for compounding to protect the public from this happening again. More FDA inspection and oversight for compounding pharmacies has been called for before. Those who fought against such oversight will now have to reconsider.

Regulations governing the development and manufacture of new drugs have gradually become far more complex and daunting over the years. So to harmonize the drug development requirements across the three main regulatory authorities, the International Conference on Harmonization (ICH), has been established to avoid unnecessary studies being conducted in animals or humans.

Will these substantial requirements be interpreted with more flexibility for the development of oligomers targeting rare diseases? That remains to be determined. The authorities are aware that the current regulations will not permit development without some flexibility, especially for rare diseases. Ongoing discussion between scientists from academia and industry with those from the regulatory authorities has been encouraged and is mediated through a think-tank, the

Oligonucleotide Safety Working Group (OSWG). Even now, the OSWG is developing consensus guidelines on various technical aspects of drug development as it applies to the new gene-patches, although such guides are not official FDA, EMA, or PMDA guidance.

The first guidance written by this think-tank with external, academic expert, and informal FDA input was published in August 2012. This guide was written to help companies and regulators understand the issues concerning the safety assessment for inhaled oligomers.

Many governments and administrations have passed orphan drug regulations in an effort to encourage development of drugs for rare diseases, with substantial success. More needs to be done; however, as the costs for drug development climb and new drug approvals decline. Against this uphill battle, several oligomer companies are now in clinical programs, studying their molecular "Band-Aids" in patients with encouraging early results.

In the next few years several of these programs are likely to lead to the final hurdle, the New Drug Application in the U.S. The FDA will review the extensive dossiers these companies have been obliged to compile. Once approved, these first few gene patch therapies will reach the marketplace.

Before explaining the drug development process in more detail, here's a quick recap of the three main agencies:

History of the U.S. FDA

The Food and Drug Administration (FDA) is an agency of the U.S. Department of Health and Human Services. It regulates anything that interacts with your body (or that of your pet's), whether you swallow it, smoke or inhale it, wear it on your skin, have it implanted inside you, or are exposed to its radiation.

The FDA is in charge of making sure that one trillion dollars worth of goods, including $275 billion in drugs, are safe for consumers.

The origin of the FDA goes back to 1883, when Harvey Washington Wiley was appointed chief chemist at the Department of Agriculture's (USDA) Division of Chemistry. He led a program of research looking into the adulteration and misbranding of food and drugs on the American market.

The USDA Division (later Bureau) of Chemistry published a ten-part series entitled "Foods and Food Adulterants" over a five-year period up to 1902. It had no power to prohibit or punish the companies responsible for the adulteration or misbranding. Wiley, however, used these findings to lobby the government. He, and others, argued that there should be uniform standards for food and drugs set by federal law. The nation's physicians, pharmacists and state regulators supported Wiley.

The public was also sympathetic following the publication of articles by Upton Sinclair and others outlining the hazards of leaving medicines unregulated. In 1906, President Theodore Roosevelt signed the Food and Drug Act into law.

This act made it illegal to transport adulterated drugs across state lines if their strength, quality or purity was not clear. The active ingredient of any medicine needed to be listed in the United States Pharmacopoeia or the National Formulary and the label on the container had to be clear. Misbranding of drugs was also declared illegal. Policing this new legislation, and examining the strength, quality and purity of drugs became the responsibility of Wiley's USDA Bureau of Chemistry.

In 1927, the Bureau of Chemistry's regulatory powers were reorganized under a new USDA body, the Food, Drug, and Insecticide organization. Then in 1930, the organization's title was changed to the Food and Drug Administration (FDA), as it remains to this day.

In the twenties, public concern was increasing about some of the drugs that were allowed under the 1906 act. The regulators and emerging consumer organizations also expressed concerns. Even the media caught on to the prevailing mood and added to the clamor for stronger regulation. A list of harmful products that had been ruled permissible under the 1906 law was published, including radioactive drinks, cosmetics that caused blindness and fraudulent claims made by drugs for diabetes and tuberculosis.

For five years, Congress procrastinated and effectively blocked any modification to the 1906 act until a tragic scandal rocked the nation in 1937. The Elixir Sulfanilamide tragedy killed over one hundred people. The drug sulfanilamide was dissolved in diethylene glycol, a toxic solvent, instead of ethanol, to form an elixir which it was claimed to be. However an elixir was defined as a medication dissolved in ethanol. The fraudulent use of the title elixir allowed the FDA to claim that the product was mislabeled and seize it. This tragedy finally forced Congress to see sense and rapidly pass a new act.

In 1938, President Franklin D. Roosevelt signed the new Food, Drug, and Cosmetic Act (FD&C Act) into law. The new act required a pre-market review of the safety of all new drugs by the FDA, significantly increasing their power to approve or veto a new drug being marketed. Companies could be punished under the new act for making false therapeutic claims in their drug's labeling. Particularly important was the fact that companies could be punished whether or not the company had been intentionally fraudulent. The new act authorized the FDA to inspect factories and, brought cosmetics and therapeutic devices under federal regulatory authority. It also set a new series of regulated standards for food. The 1938 FD&C Act remains the central foundation of today's FDA regulatory oversight.

Soon after passage of the 1938 Act, the FDA began to designate certain drugs as safe for use only under the supervision of a medical professional. Prescription-only drugs became a designation in the 1951 Durham-Humphrey Amendment. Over the next quarter century, the FDA reviewed 13,000 new drug applications (NDAs), although much of it's attention was focused on amphetamine and barbiturate abuse.

In 1959, further congressional hearings into concerns about pharmaceutical industry practices were held. Many thought that some promoted drugs were too expensive and had dubious claims of benefit. But as with the earlier calls for stricter regulation, any new legislation expanding the FDA's powers was strongly opposed by vested interests.

Once again it took a tragedy to force politicians to act.

Although thalidomide had been blocked by the FDA from release in the U.S., it was marketed in Europe with tragic results. I can remember when English babies were born with deformed limbs after their mothers took thalidomide, which was marketed for treatment of "morning sickness" in early pregnancy. Routine ultrasound scanning had not then been established and thus the deformities were not detected until the first babies were born. Thalidomide was estimated to have affected up to 20,000 babies before it was withdrawn in 1961.

The thalidomide tragedy in Europe led to the passage of important legislation in the U.S. In 1962, a watershed moment in FDA history took place. An amendment to the FD&C act was passed. Substantial evidence of efficacy for any claim put forward was now required as part of any new drug application.

This was in addition to the existing requirement for pre-marketing demonstration of safety.

Substantial evidence of safety in animals is needed before the FDA will allow even very small single doses of a drug to be given to humans. A large body of preliminary toxicological data is therefore common as part of the investigational new drug (IND) application that the FDA reviews before any clinical study in humans can begin.

The 1962 Amendment marked the start of the FDA approval process as we now know it today. It also required that drugs approved between 1938 and 1962 be reviewed by the FDA for evidence of efficacy. When that efficacy was not satisfactorily demonstrated, the offending drug was withdrawn from the market.

The amendment also restricted advertising to FDA-approved indications, and expanded FDA powers to inspect drug manufacturing facilities.

Due to these requirements, it took longer to develop a drug, which shortened the time a drug could be sold before its patent expired. Once a drug is out of patent, anyone can manufacture and sell a generic version of the same drug, without performing any additional research. Thus generic manufacturers do not have to work for a decade developing a huge dossier of data, nor spend the money required to do so. With no development costs, they can charge for just the cost of manufacturing and their profit. That's why generic drugs cost so much less than brand-name drugs. To try and match these generic drug prices, the original brand's price often tumbles when its patent expires, so it becomes far less profitable.

To compensate for this, the Hatch-Waxman Act of 1984 was passed. This bill extended the amount of time a drug manufacturer could hold a patent on a drug before the generic manufacturers could enter the market.

In the 1980s, the AIDS epidemic struck. New drugs were needed and HIV activist organizations expressed concerns about the time it took for the FDA to review and approve these vital drugs. Large protests were staged, including a confrontational one in October 1988 at the FDA campus resulting in nearly 180 arrests. By 1990, it was estimated that thousands of lives were lost each year due to delays in approval and marketing of drugs for cancer and AIDS.

In 1987, the FDA introduced Treatment INDs to allow promising new drugs to be made available to desperately ill patients as early in the drug development process as possible, once there is preliminary evidence of drug efficacy and the drug is intended to treat a serious or life-threatening disease, or if there is no alternative drug or therapy available. Treatment INDs are made available to doctors and their patients before general marketing begins, typically during phase 3 studies. They also allow the manufacturer and the FDA to obtain additional data on the drug's safety and effectiveness.

Treatment INDs are rare. In the first 12 years only 39 such applications have been approved, of which 13 were for cancer and 11 were for HIV/AIDS. The accelerated approval rules were further expanded and codified in 1992.

All of the initial drugs approved for the treatment of HIV/AIDS were approved through accelerated approval mechanisms. For example, a treatment IND was issued for the first HIV drug, AZT, in 1985, and approval was granted just two years later in 1987. Three of the first five drugs targeting HIV were approved in the U.S. before they were approved in any other country.

The Critical Path Initiative, launched in 2004, is the FDA's effort to stimulate and facilitate a national focus on modernizing how FDA-regulated products are developed, evaluated, and manufactured. Nonetheless, criticism of the time it takes the FDA to review and approve drugs continues. The AIDS crisis created political efforts to streamline the approval process, but these limited reforms were targeted for AIDS drugs, not the broader market. This led to the call for more enduring reforms that would allow patients to have access to drugs that have passed the first round of clinical trials. These would be patients suffering from rare and lethal diseases, and treatment would be under the care of doctors.

Oligomers in development for rare diseases are currently reviewed in the same way as other new drugs, and thus have required as much data to support their safety, especially toxicological data, as conventional drugs. When their clinical development plans advance, the number of patients with each rare disease, or each subset with any particular genetic variation, will be insufficient to meet the high hurdles that all drugs are expected to surpass.

The Center for Drug Evaluation and Research (CDER) has different requirements for the three main types of drug products: new drugs, generic drugs and over-the-counter drugs. A drug is considered "new" if it is made by a different manufacturer, uses different excipients or inactive ingredients, is used for a different purpose, or undergoes any substantial change. The most rigorous requirements apply to "new molecular entities" (NMEs): drugs that are not based on existing medications. All oligomers currently in development fall in this category and will receive extensive assessment before FDA approval in the NDA process.

In 2006, at the request of Congress, a committee was appointed by the Institute of Medicine to review pharmaceutical safety regulation in the U.S. It found major deficiencies in the current FDA system for ensuring the safety of marketed drugs and called for an increase in the regulatory powers, funding, and independence of the FDA. Some of the committee's recommendations were incorporated into the Food and Drug Administration Act, which was signed into law in 2007. This law requires that the FDA review new drugs within ten months. It has been a successful piece of legislation, more than doubling the proportion of NDAs the FDA reviews within one year to 95% of those submitted. This has led to more companies submitting their NDAs to the FDA and aiming for launch in the U.S. first.

The FDA collects fees for the review of all NDAs, thus the Food and Drug Administration Act has generated more revenue for Uncle Sam from these.

The Safety of Drugs for Children

Prior to the 1990s, only twenty percent of all drugs prescribed for children had been tested for safety and efficacy in a pediatric population. This became a major concern of pediatricians as evidence accumulated that the physiological response of children to many drugs differed significantly from those seen in adults. For many drugs, children represented such a small proportion of the total potential market that such testing would not be cost-effective. There were also concerns about the feasibility and ethics of children providing informed consent. In addition, increased governmental and institutional hurdles for these clinical trials were encountered, as well as greater concerns about liability. Thus, for decades, most medicines prescribed to children were done so in an "off-label" manner, with dosages extrapolated from adult data through body weight and body-surface-area calculations.

After several initiatives proved unsuccessful at stimulating more widespread pediatric clinical studies, Congress used the 1997 Food and Drug Administration Modernization Act (FDAMA) to pass incentives which gave a six-month patent term extension to pharmaceutical manufacturers on new drugs submitted with pediatric trial data.

In a 2001 report, the General Accounting Office of the U.S. government confirmed that this law had been successful. Before 1997, up to eighty percent of drug labels had inadequate pediatric data. Within four years, the FDA had received 188 requests for the marketing extension allowable under FDAMA. These requests included data from 414 studies covering 23,200 children. New drugs were the subject of 33 of these requests, while 155 applications concerned drugs already approved but lacking pediatric data.

Most recently, in the Pediatric Research Equity Act of 2003, Congress codified the FDA's authority to mandate manufacturer-sponsored pediatric drug trials as a "last resort" if incentives and publicly funded mechanisms proved inadequate. Several of the oligomers currently in advanced clinical development are for pediatric diseases.

History of the European Medicines Agency

The European Medicines Agency (EMA) was, until 2004, known as European Agency for the Evaluation of Medicinal Products (EMEA). The EMA is the pharmaceutical regulatory body of the European Union (EU). It's based in London. Before the EMEA was established, each country in Europe relied on its own national regulatory authority to regulate drug approvals. Although the national authorities have not been disbanded they now work with the EMA, often in a sort of subcontractor role. The EMEA was born after more than seven years of negotiations among EU governments and replaced the Committee for Proprietary Medicinal Products (CPMP) and the Committee for Veterinary Medicinal Products. Both of these committees were reborn as the core scientific advisory committees within the newly formed EMEA.

Roughly parallel to the U.S. FDA, but without FDA-style centralization, the EMA was originally set up in 1995 with EU and pharmaceutical industry funding, as well as indirect subsidy from member states. The EMA is an attempt to harmonize (but not replace) the work of existing national European medicine and regulatory bodies and thereby reduce the $350 million annual cost drug companies incurred by having to win separate approvals from each member state. It was also hoped that the EMA's creation would eliminate the protectionist tendencies of some states unwilling to approve new drugs manufactured by companies in other countries that might compete with domestic drug companies. The main responsibility and mission of the EMA is to coordinate the scientific resources of the 27 EU Member States, with a view to providing European citizens with high quality, safe, and effective medicines for humans and animals and, at the same time, to advance towards a single market for medicines. The European Union is currently the source of about one-third of the new drugs brought onto the world market each year.

The EMA is run by a management board that provides administrative oversight. It is responsible for approval of budgets and plans, and selection of the executive director. The board includes one representative from each of the 27 member states (Figure 9.1), two representatives of the European Commission, two representatives of the European Parliament, two representatives of patients' organizations, one representative of doctors' organizations and one representative of veterinarians' organizations. The EMA works through a network of roughly 4500 EU experts to decentralize its scientific assessment of medicines and draws on resources from over forty National Competent Authorities (NCAs) from EU member states.

Companies can submit a single application to the agency to obtain a centralized approval valid in all EU and European Free Trade Association states (including Iceland, Liechtenstein and Norway). The centralized procedure is compulsory for all medicines derived from biotechnology and other high-tech processes, as well as for human medicines for the treatment of HIV/AIDS, cancer, diabetes, neuro-degenerative diseases, auto-immune and other immune dysfunctions, and viral diseases. The therapeutic oligomers for rare diseases will be reviewed by this centralized procedure in due course.

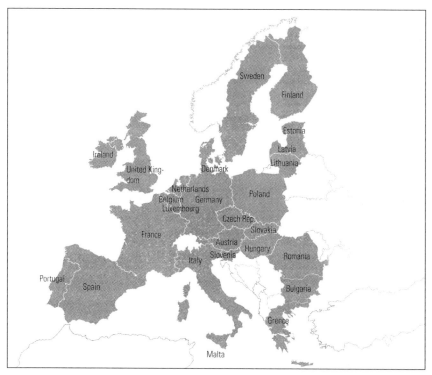

Figure 9.1. The 27 EU Member states. Note Switzerland and Norway are not EU Member States.

A single centralized marketing authorization application (MAA) is submitted to the EMA and a single evaluation is carried out by the Committee for Medicinal Products for Human Use (CHMP). If the committee approves the drug, it's virtually guaranteed that the European Commission will approve it for sale throughout the whole of the EU.

The CHMP is obliged by the Regulations to reach decisions within 210 days, although the clock is stopped when the applicant company is asked for clarification or further supporting data. This compares favorably with the average of 500 days taken by the FDA.

The Pediatric Committee (PDCO) deals with the implementation of the 2007 pediatric legislation which requires all new MAAs, or variations to existing authorizations, to either include data from pediatric studies (previously agreed with the PDCO), or to have received a waiver or a deferral for these studies from the PDCO. So, the EMA like the FDA is keen to ensure that new drugs will be made available for children and that pediatric data will be submitted as part of the MAA.

History of the Japanese PMDA

In Japan, the Ministry of Health, Labor, and Welfare establishes drug regulations. It was formed by the merger of the former Ministry of Health and Welfare and the Ministry of Labor, and began accepting submissions for new product approvals in July 2001.

Following the Reorganization and Rationalization Plan for Special Public Corporations that was approved in a Cabinet meeting in 2001, the Pharmaceuticals and Medical Devices Agency (PMDA) was established and came into service on April 1, 2004, the Japanese counterpart to FDA and EMA. The services of the Pharmaceuticals and Medical Devices Evaluation Center of the National Institute of Health Sciences, the Organization for Pharmaceutical Safety and Research, and part of the Japan Association for the Advancement of Medical Equipment were consolidated under the Law that established the PMDA.

The PMDA has three main areas of activity: Drug and Medical Device review, post-marketing safety and compensation for adverse drug effects. As with FDA and EMA, the PMDA has numerous departments and divisions.

International Conference on Harmonization

It became apparent during the 1960s, 70s and 80s that different requirements for drug development were being imposed on global pharmaceutical companies by the three main regulatory authorities. This led to inefficiency, some unnecessary duplication, greater expense, and delay in new drugs being registered in some markets. Harmonization of regulatory requirements was pioneered by the European Community (EC), in the 1980s, as the EC moved towards the development of a single market in Europe for pharmaceuticals.

The success achieved in Europe demonstrated that harmonization was feasible. At the same time there were bilateral discussions between Europe, Japan and the U.S. on possibilities for wider harmonization. At the 1989 World Health Organization (WHO) Conference of Drug Regulatory Authorities in Paris, specific planning for action started. Soon afterwards, the authorities approached the International Federation of Pharmaceutical Manufacturers and Associations to discuss a joint regulatory-industry initiative on international harmonization, and ICH was conceived.

The birth of ICH took place at a meeting in April 1990, hosted by the European Federation of Pharmaceutical Industries and Associations in Brussels. Representatives of the regulatory agencies and industry associations of Europe, Japan and the U.S. met, primarily, to plan an International Conference but the meeting also discussed the wider implications and terms of reference of ICH. It has evolved since its inception through its Global Cooperation Group, to respond to the increasingly global face of drug development. ICH's mission is to achieve greater harmonization to ensure that safe, effective, and high quality medicines are developed and registered in the most resource-efficient manner.

Other countries, outside the original U.S., European and Japanese founders of ICH, are increasingly getting involved in ICH developments, bringing harmonization of regulatory requirements to an ever wider market. Authorities such as Health Canada, Australia's Therapeutic Goods Administration and New Zealand's Medsafe are closely aligned with the principals and practice of ICH. India, China and

Brazil are all increasingly adopting FDA-like structures and operating practices in a bid to speed up access to new drugs in their domains. This is good news for pharmaceutical and biotech companies and for the patients suffering from rare diseases, their families and the healthcare professionals caring for them.

The Regulatory Authorities and Oligomers

In September 2009, AVI BioPharma (now Sarepta Therapeutics), and the other companies working on four specific neuromuscular diseases, were invited by TreatNMD to a preliminary discussion which they hosted at the EMA in London. At the time I was chief medical officer for AVI and we had an ongoing clinical study at London's Great Ormond Street Hospital for Sick Children and the University of Newcastle in the UK.

TreatNMD (treat neuromuscular disease, www.treat-nmd.eu/about/network/) is a European network of academics, clinicians, charities and industry employees seeking ways to accelerate the development of new therapies in neuromuscular disease. The meeting aimed to bring regulators, academia, advocacy groups and industry together to discuss the issues raised by the development of therapeutic oligomers for the four lethal neuromuscular diseases: Duchenne muscular dystrophy (DMD), Spinal Muscular Atrophy (SMA), Amyotrophic Lateral Sclerosis (ALS) and Myotonic Dystrophy (MD). Each of these diseases is being tackled by disparate teams of scientists, researchers and companies scattered around the world. I was asked to present some of the emerging data with AVI-4658 in DMD, that I was responsible for overseeing, and other companies and academics presented data they had generated.

The outcome of, and hope generated at, this meeting was subsequently published (Muntoni. Neuromusc Dis 2010) and was then followed by a second meeting hosted by the U.S. National Institutes of Health (NIH) in Washington DC in October 2010. FDA attendance at this second meeting was much greater, with numerous staff from the Office of Orphan Product Development attending [http://www.fda.gov/AboutFDA/CentersOffices/OC/OfficeofScienceandHealth Coordination/OfficeofOrphanProductDevelopment/default.htm].

I was invited to sit on one of several panels at this second meeting that discussed the obstacles to successful development of oligomers and possible solutions to those problems. At both of these meetings, all parties agreed that the current regulations would need more flexible interpretation to allow drugs to be developed for very small populations of patients, in some cases less than one hundred. It was left for industry to prompt the agencies to consider the issues by engaging in dialogue early, repeatedly and frequently. Both the EMA and FDA have encouraged companies to approach them for advice to help design clinical studies and both have formal mechanisms for that advice to be requested and provided.

The regulations are there for a purpose, to safeguard the public. But while the long path to drug marketing approval has historically been the safe and cautious way to test new chemical entities, should the same path be adopted for rare diseases? The large numbers of patients required for today's conventional safety testing will never be available for any one rare disease.

An interesting analogy was made at the TreatNMD/EMA meeting by the Dutch DMD Parent Project organization. "Society expects there to be traffic laws and for all cars to obey a restricted speed limit in towns. That makes it safer for other drivers, cyclists and pedestrians. But emergency vehicles, driven by carefully trained drivers, are given special dispensation to exceed these limits when rushing to or from an emergency. Why cannot we have a similar "fast track" process for drugs intended to treat rare diseases, especially those previously undruggable, currently untreatable and universally lethal?"

The good news is that the regulatory authorities do indeed have some "fast track" regulations, and perhaps yet faster paths to approval can and will be agreed over the next few years as the oligomers in development start to build some traction.

Current Path to Approval for a New Drug

People wonder why it takes so long to get a new drug to market. Sometimes press releases from an early research project suggesting possible future benefit from a drug may give the misleading impression that the drug will be available within days, weeks, or months. That is regrettable, as drug development is already very complex, highly regulated, subject to detailed and lengthy review by the regulatory agencies, and often only follows years of careful clinical research. That clinical research involves testing of the new drug in hundreds, sometimes thousands of patients with the disease of interest.

Here are the complicated steps that a new drug, from a new class, must go through before the dossier of results can be submitted to the FDA, EMA or PMDA for approval:

1. Drug Discovery

First a disease is identified that needs treatment. Understanding how the disease starts and what causes it is vital before a new drug can be sought to solve that problem. Then a series of chemicals may be investigated in the laboratory to see which, if any, may be effective in that disease. Currently much of that drug design looks at a target receptor that is key to how the disease affects people. Hopefully, the drug being sought will bind to that receptor and block it, or stimulate it. For the oligomers, which share a string of building blocks of synthetic nucleotides, this step can be skipped.

2. Basic Research

Long before a drug goes anywhere near a patient, early research must determine that it works in the test tube. For the oligomers, several patches may be tested to find the one that binds best to the target area of the faulty RNA. It is known, for instance that certain areas of pre-messenger RNA have sections that when read will initiate splicing, so called enhancer sites. These areas, and those immediately adjacent, are the focus of attention when alternative splicing needs to be triggered. Nowadays experiments can be run on several different patches at the same time to identify, in the laboratory, which seems to be the most efficient. The best result leads to that particular sequence being selected as the "drug candidate."

The drug candidate in the test tube then needs to be tested in living cells to see if it does indeed do what is required of it. On passing this hurdle, if there are animal models of the disease, the drug will be tested in a whole live animal. It is important to confirm that the drug will indeed get into the cells and work.

3. Toxicology Studies in Animals

Next comes a toxicology program, using animals, to investigate how safe a drug is, long before it goes anywhere near a human. While it is regrettable that animals need to be used in these experiments, computer modeling is just not sophisticated enough to be able to predict and replicate how a whole animal, especially a mammal, will respond to a new drug.

Laboratory scientists are acutely aware of the issues and ethics of drug testing in animals and the vast majority of this early work is conducted under closely monitored conditions to minimize any suffering to the animals involved. Much of the early research for many drugs, but especially the new oligomers, is conducted in mice. These mice have often been specially bred for these experiments. Sometimes they have a mouse equivalent of the human disease, as in DMD. In other cases, sometimes a human gene is bred into the mice so that the effect of a new drug for human disease can be tested on the human gene, in the humanized mouse.

The toxicology testing program in animals is a complex process that often takes several years.

An early step is to assess the amount of a drug that is absorbed into the body of a mammal (especially if is given by mouth). When given directly by intravenous injection, this amount is assumed to be 100% of the dose. The researchers then try to determine where this dose is distributed and in which organs it accumulates. This will help to decide which organs should be more carefully examined in the general toxicology studies.

There are four key steps to predicting how a drug will behave in humans, which can easily be remembered using the acronym ADME:

A. Absorption: How much of a new drug is absorbed in to the body

D. Distribution: Where the drug then distributes to and what levels it accumulates to in the various tissues

M. Metabolism: Where and how the new drug is metabolized, for instance by the liver, and understanding what products the drug breaks up into

E. Elimination: How are the parent molecule and/or its metabolites eliminated

Another early step in the preclinical testing is a series of safety pharmacology studies, usually single dose. These look at specific organ systems in much greater depth than is undertaken in the routine toxi-cology testing. The cardiovascular, respiratory, and the neurological systems are usually the focus of these studies. Special studies may also be needed either before or during human testing to look at the effect of the new drug on cardiac conduction and other organ systems.

Generally, the FDA requires data on safety for a new drug to be generated in two species before human testing can commence. For most drugs one rodent, mouse or rat, and one larger species are needed. In many cases, specially bred beagle dogs, are the second species, but for oligomers, most companies choose small monkeys. Since they are genetically and physiologically closer to humans, their data may be more accurate at predicting safety in humans.

The program usually starts off in mammals of one species to determine the maximum tolerated dose (MTD). After the tolerability of a single dose has been determined, multiple doses will be tested, administered in the same way as it will be later in humans. The most common ways drugs are given are intravenously, orally or by inhalation, but there are other routes including subcutaneous or intramuscular injection. These chronic dosing studies are expected to identify the dose at which there are no side effects, called the "no adverse effect level" (NOAEL). The gap between the NOAEL and the MTD gives an indication of a drug's safety. The wider the gap, the safer the drug is expected to be in subsequent human testing.

The toxicology program, especially the crucial multiple dose studies lasting for 14, 28, or 90 days must be conducted under very carefully controlled conditions. These programs are conducted in special facili-ties that have been carefully designed to control the environment and allow careful observation of the animals. These facilities may at any time be inspected by the company whose drug is being studied, by an auditor on behalf of the company, or by one or other of the regulatory authorities. The facilities also have to follow rules established by special animal use committees who oversee all animal experiments. This is to ensure that animals do not suffer unnecessarily in the quest to develop safer, more effective drugs for human use.

The FDA expects companies to take a fraction of NOAEL dose, ranging from as little as one percent to as much as five percent, as the starting dose in subsequent first-time-in-human single dose testing.

In addition to the data provided to enable human testing to begin, other more specialized toxicology studies may be required. Reproductive toxicology will be required for any drug that is being developed for possible use during pregnancy. Studies of juvenile animals are required if the drug is intended for children, and most drugs that are intended for chronic use in humans have to undergo longer term chronic testing, often up to nine months duration in two species. Another expensive study to conduct is the two-year carcinogenicity trial to determine if the drug causes cancer in animals. This is often irrespective of whether the early gene-toxicity showed any likelihood of damage to animal genes even at extremely high doses in the test tube. And this is by no means a comprehensive list of all the studies that may be required. Some of the work can be delayed, especially the nine months of chronic dosing and the carcinogenicity study, until early human results have been obtained. If single doses of the drug are not well tolerated by humans, then longer term testing will not be allowed, so these longer term studies in animals are not needed.

4. Chemistry, Manufacturing and Controls (CMC)

All drugs approved by the FDA have to pass stringent standards for purity and quality. The quality of a new drug and its purity and stability during storage and shipping, commonly known as the shelf life, must be assured before it can be tested in humans. The paper trail for a new drug has to go back to the very earliest ingredients that have been used to make the raw materials for even the first step in what, for oligomers, is a series of many complex steps. At each step, the manufacturing process has to be carefully documented and explained. Records must be reviewed that show the materials adhere to very tight specifications for stability and purity. The final product, intended for human use in the first set of safety studies has to have records that stretch back to the first basic ingredients. And they must be available for inspection and approval by the FDA.

The final product, the active pharmaceutical ingredient (API), has to be stored without degrading for periods of time considerably longer than those likely to be encountered in early clinical testing. In addition, the API, in its packaging, must be exposed to extremes of both temperature and humidity and yet remain pure and potent.

Most of the oligomers in development will be dry powders or solutions in glass vials with rubber stoppers. Other medicines use a variety of containers that you're probably familiar with, including foil-backed blister packs or small screw-top bottles for pills, plastic ampules for liquid solutions, and metal canisters for inhaled drugs. These systems have to be studied to ensure that the material they are made of does not leak into the medicines. In addition, the medicine must not get absorbed onto the container's walls.

This basic quality data is a vital part of the information required before any human testing can take place. As a drug goes through clinical testing in humans, the clinical studies get longer as the program advances. And these clinical studies will be conducted in patients over a wider geographical area. Thus CMC data generation continues to evolve in parallel to the clinical work during the long process from bench top to bedside. By the time a drug has completed a clinical development program, the CMC data fills many gigabytes of hard disc space. Also, the manufacturing process is refined and improved as development proceeds. But once clinical testing reaches its last step, the manufacturing process must be finalized. From then on it cannot be changed. This even includes the color of the ink on a label, for fear that a new pigment may leak in through the walls of the drug container and affect the purity of a compound that was tested.

5. Clinical Studies – in Humans

Once animal testing has provided sufficient safety data to enable human testing, an investigational new drug (IND) application is prepared and submitted to the FDA. There is an equivalent dossier, an Investigational Medicinal Product Dossier in Europe. These dossiers and their submission are a key landmark in the life of any company, but especially any small company. All the previous research, quality and animal toxicology data must be submitted. A protocol for the proposed first human study is also included. In the U.S., the FDA has a stipulated thirty days to review all this information and decide if the data is sufficient to allow the proposed human study to proceed. If the FDA is not satisfied, which sometimes happens, they impose a "clinical hold" on the program until the deficiencies have been addressed.

Human research is often divided into three phases:

Phase I: Single dose and then short term multiple-dose testing is often undertaken in otherwise healthy adult volunteers. The starting dose is a fraction of the NOAEL, discovered in animal trials, ranging from as little as one to five percent.

Frequently, an independent data safety monitoring board, or DSMB, will review the information from each step before permission is granted to escalate to a higher dose. The aim is to reach a dose where troubling side effects may start to appear, which is called "dose limiting toxicity." This dose needs to be well above what the expected effective dose of the drug is, giving it a wide safety margin. Some drugs continue with testing even when this safety margin is rather narrow.

This phase may involve a small number of subjects, usually less than one hundred. In addition to very careful observation of all bodily functions, blood samples may be taken at frequent intervals over a period of hours or days after dosing to see how the volunteers eliminate the drug from the blood stream. This is the science of pharmacokinetics, what the body does to the drug. The close observation, often combined with intensive monitoring of some or all bodily systems, is the companion science of pharmacodynamics, what the drug does to the body.

New cancer drugs usually skip this phase because even at a low dose they will cause unpleasant side effects in human volunteers. Thus the early single and then multiple dose testing studies are conventionally conducted in small numbers of cancer patients.

The initial safety testing of the new oligomers will be done in patients with the specific disease they target, rather than healthy volunteers. The oligomers will patch the messenger RNA that is faulty by binding to a tiny section of it. If they were given to normal volunteers, they would bind to the same message that might have adverse consequences.

There are lots of questions. In August 2012, the first of several discussion papers was published in Nucleic Acid Therapeutics (NAT) by one of the subcommittees of the Oligonucleotide Safety Working Group (OSWG). The paper summarized the opinions of academic and industrial researchers and clinicians about how the safety of inhaled oligomers should be assessed.

The OSWG is a loosely knit think tank of over one hundred scientists from academia, industry and regulatory agencies, for which I act as volunteer publications coordinator. We are keen to develop guidelines about how best to assess the safety of these exciting new drugs in both animals and humans. Several more guidelines developed by various subgroups focusing on different areas of testing – mainly preclinical (i.e. before the oligomers are given to humans) are in development. In some cases the papers have been submitted to scientific journals for publication and over the coming years more debate and discussion will occur. Hopefully, consensus will emerge.

New gene patches being developed to block lethal viruses don't need to skip phase I. Outbreaks of Ebola or Marburg hemorrhagic fever are likely to occur in populations where at least some of those infected will be otherwise healthy adults. The viral mRNA is unique to the virus and there is no identical message within the normal human genome. Thus phase I testing of the new antiviral translation suppressing oligomers (TSO) has been conducted in healthy volunteers.

Phase II: In phase II, different doses of the drug and different regimens such as once or twice daily, will be tested. In the case of oligomers, a lesser frequency may be tested, maybe once a week or less. Different formulations may also be tried and if the drug is given intravenously, different speeds of injection, ranging from a slow drip that takes over 12 hours to an injection that takes two minutes. This phase is conducted to confirm that the drug does works, and what doses it works at.

If the drug is designed to treat hypertension, lowering of the blood pressure is desired. How much is the blood pressure lowered? How soon after taking the drug? How long does the lowering affect last after each dose? All of these questions, and many more, need to be answered in this phase.

For many diseases, such as high blood pressure, methods for monitoring the effect, the recording of blood pressure, have been available for many years, and doctors and staff are familiar with how to record measurements. For rare diseases that is not always the case.

In the case of Duchenne muscular dystrophy (DMD), for example, there is no history of testing even mildly effective drugs and no experience with how to monitor beneficial effects. In this case, the phase II experiment measures different possible effects and explores which benefit is easiest to measure. It then looks at how much that measure changes in patients, and for how long. Because the clinical benefit of these new medicines may take weeks or even months to become apparent, doctors are looking for biomarkers, a biological effect that is easier to measure that will predict clinical benefit. For DMD, the ultimate clinical benefit is a longer life, but that may take up to thirty years to prove. Shorter term, the ability of the new oligomers to slow the loss of muscle function, halt decline or even restore muscle function would be an ideal marker to follow.

The problem is that boys with DMD have been without dystrophin in their muscles since birth. Is the new appearance of dystrophin in their muscles ten years down the road going to translate into an immediate clinical benefit, as measured by the distance they can walk in six minutes? That experiment has now been conducted by both companies working with DMD splice switching oligomers. Both Pronsena and Sarepta believe the answer is yes.

What is easier to demonstrate is the appearance of new dystrophin in the muscles of these boys, through the use of tissue biopsies. This may become a biomarker for other effective DMD oligomers in the future, should the levels of the novel dystrophin found prove to correlate with subsequent substantial clinical benefit.

One other note: In the case of all drugs (with the exception of those for cancer and oligomers), phase I is performed in healthy volunteers.

Phase II is conducted in patients who are ill with the disease for which the drug is intended.

A phase II program can be complex with multiple studies conducted over a period of several years. This is the phase where other specialized studies may need to be conducted: interaction with other drugs, possible effects on the electrical activity in the heart, and how well the drug works in patients who have another disease as well. These studies are usually longer than phase I and involve more subjects. Tens or even hundreds of patients are often studied in each phase II trial.

Phase III: Once an efficacy signal has been detected in phase II, there is often a meeting between the sponsoring company and the FDA. It is important at this meeting to agree on the signal, the benefit of the drug being tested, and the design of a pair of pivotal studies to confirm its beneficial effect. Thus phase III is the confirmatory phase of drug development which seeks to provide the pivotal data on which its approval will be based.

Depending on the disease being studied, the phase III program could be just this single pair of studies. But sometimes the company wants to prove benefit in more than one indication, or more than one type of patient. Depending on how different the types of patients are, the pair of studies may need to be analyzed in a more complicated way, either analyzing them by subset, or conducting additional, different studies. This phase is much larger, with several hundred to sometimes thousands of patients enrolled in a study. There are dozens, even hundreds of investigational centers, spread across many continents and countries. They are extremely expensive. An individual phase III study may cost anywhere from ten million to one hundred million dollars to conduct, and take many years to set up, execute and analyze. This is true even if the actual study period is only a few weeks.

The most likely oligomer to be reviewed next, now that mipomersen has been approved, is the Prosensa DMD drug, PRO051, which is being supported by GlaxoSmithKline. A phase III study of 180 Duchenne boys, which now appears to have fully enrolled, is currently ongoing at the time of this writing.

To avoid bias, phase III studies are often double blind and placebo controlled. That means that neither the doctors nor their staff, nor the volunteers with the disease know if they are receiving active drug or a placebo. Even rare disease drugs may be compared against a placebo, as is the case for PRO051. Such placebo controlled testing is regarded as the gold standard of drug study design.

At all phases of the clinical program, subjects, be they healthy volunteers or patients with mild, moderate or severe disease, must participate in the research voluntarily. Since the Geneva conventions after the Second World War, a process called informed consent has been enforced. Here the benefits and risks of the research has to be explained to and understood by the subjects. They must sign a voluntary agreement that states there has been no coercion. This consent process is a vital step before any study–related procedure can be conducted.

Investigational Review Boards/Ethics Committees

Another key protection that has been built into clinical research is the establishment of Investigational Review Boards (IRBs) in the U.S. In other parts of the world they are called "ethics committees," but they have the same function. These committees are composed of doctors, attorneys, ethicists, and lay people who are not affiliated in any way with the company conducting the research, nor the investigational sites where the research is being executed. The members of the ethics committee may not be associated with any of the regulatory authorities. The IRB has the responsibility of ensuring that the research is conducted ethically and responsibly by all concerned. They review the language in the consent form which explains what is proposed to confirm that the explanation is understandable to the subjects.

Clinical Investigator Brochure

An important document is the Clinical Investigator Brochure (CIB, or just IB). It serves as a reference manual for the doctors in charge of supervising dosing throughout the clinical program. For the phase 1 studies, it summarizes the work carried out in animals as well as basic information about the disease for which the new drug is being tested. As the clinical program proceeds, the CIB is updated at least once a year.

Post-Approval Monitoring

FDA interest in drugs does not end however when a drug is approved. After NDA approval, the sponsor must review and report every ordinary adverse patient drug experience it learns of, at least quarterly. Unexpected serious and fatal adverse drug events must be reported within 15 days.

The FDA also receives "spontaneous reports" about possible adverse drug events through its MedWatch program. These voluntary reports are received directly from consumers and health professionals. This program has been the primary tool of post- market safety surveillance.

Vioxx, as discussed in Chapter 4, is a non-steroidal anti-inflammatory drug that was approved in the U.S. in 1999. However, several subsequent studies suggested that Vioxx might increase the risk of fatal heart attacks. In 2004, these fears were confirmed, leading to its much publicized, voluntary removal from the market by Merck.

More recently, the case of Avandia, a diabetes drug manufactured by GlaxoSmithKline, generated controversy. In June 2010, a retrospective study of 227,571 elderly American patients, comparing Avandia to other similar U.S. diabetes drugs was published. The authors concluded that Avandia was associated with "an increased risk of stroke, heart failure, and all-cause mortality." Based on the study, only sixty patients needed to be treated with Avandia for one to come to harm.

In March 2011, a meta-analysis of observational studies, involving 810,000 patients, provided more evidence that Avandia was associated with a higher risk of heart failure, myocardial infarction and death than a similar drug, pioglitazone. Other reports comparing Avandia to other diabetes drugs (including the 2009 RECORD study published in the Lancet) were less unfavorable and were reviewed by an FDA panel. The controversy led to the FDA requiring stricter prescribing rules and patient warnings as well as calls for a general increase in the amount of pre- and post- approval safety data.

As a result of these highly publicized cases, FDA requirements for post-marketing risk management are increasing. As a condition of approval, a sponsor may be required to conduct additional clinical trials, called Phase IV trials. The FDA is increasingly requiring risk management plans for drugs as part of a development program that may call for additional studies, restrictions, or safety surveillance activities.

High profile public and scientific debates continue about whether new drugs should be evaluated on the basis of their absolute safety, or on their safety relative to existing treatments. The FDA is in an unenviable position. The public wants access to effective medicines as quickly as possible, yet serious safety concerns may not be detected by current standard development programs. What they may require is many thousands of patient-years of treatment. These conflicting requirements are impossible to resolve especially for drugs being developed for rare diseases.

Summary

The big three Regulatory Authorities, FDA, EMA, and PMDA, have all grown and evolved over recent decades. They are now large organizations responsible for approving the marketing of effective and safe drugs that have been manufactured to adequate levels of quality. Globalization of pharmaceutical development and approval has led to many national authorities in other countries taking their lead from the FDA.

Current requirements for registration of a new drug throughout the world have grown dramatically over the last half-century. Regulation was introduced to protect the public from the unscrupulous few, in this case doctors and pharmaceutical manufacturers. More recently, there has been additional scientific assessment of new drugs and increasing sophistication, as well as beneficial harmonization of the regulatory authorities. The path to approval for a new drug is now harder than ever, and discourages many companies. Between 2007 and 2009, thirty percent of all newly marketed medicines were modifications of already approved drugs. For instance, old drugs were reformulated and given as an injection instead of a tablet, or vice versa. Or old drugs were modified for a new indication but borrowed the safety record of the original drug. Many companies and their investors feel that it is a safer investment to wring more life out of old approved drugs than to try and develop new ones.

How will the high hurdles be overcome by the new wave of oligomers? How many patients with any one rare disease can these new drugs can be tested on? The answers will be provided over the next few years if the oligomers in development live up to their early promise.

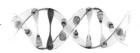

Chapter Ten

The Pharmacy of the Future

While personalized medicine has clear medical benefits, the concept of deliberately narrowing the target markets of drugs in development creates a dilemma for pharmaceutical developers.

The traditional pharmaceutical companies will need to rely more on innovation as revenue models fueled by a few billion-dollar blockbuster drugs are no longer relevant. Eventually, all companies will need to rely on a broader array of smaller market drugs to fill their product portfolios. Instead of economy of manufacturing for a single drug, companies will need to develop broader economic models involving many individual oligomers – or conventional small molecule drugs. In addition, companies focused on rare and lethal diseases will have to balance the cost of the development of each of their new personalized drugs with the much smaller, more focused target audience.

Should the individual patients or their healthcare insurance bear the cost of these new therapies? I anticipate that some of the new oligomers will cost $250,000/year or even more. Or should the cost of these drugs for a few be spread across society as a whole? Whoever pays, it should be noted that their cost may be considerably less than the cost of not having adequate, safe treatment. That cost is currently born by the patients, their family, their healthcare insurance systems, and by society. The cost of caring for a patient slowly dying from a lethal genetic disorder may far exceed the cost of a new treatment – in terms of both healthcare dollars and impact on the patient's family, community, and the economy.

Speed to market will be even more important than today where millions of dollars may be lost if a new drug is delayed by a few weeks from being approved. In the future, delay in a drug gaining approval will not only affect the company coffers, but in the case of rare disease treatments, it may cost patients their lives.

The regulatory agencies are aware of the dilemma they face. They are keen not to delay a lifesaving medicine from reaching the market. At the same time, though, they must be sufficiently confident that the benefits of the drug outweigh the risk. Has the sponsor presented enough data to allow that informed decision to be made?

That is one good reason for the companies developing drugs for rare diseases, to be in frequent and detailed dialogue with the FDA. Unfortunately, the FDA, as with many important regulatory agencies, has suffered cutbacks and layoffs, while the workload has become heavier and more complex for the remaining staff. In addition, if the agency is too approachable there will be a fear of collusion with the drug companies and critical voices will be raised by agency watchers.

A more flexible regulatory authority review is already enshrined in the orphan drug regulations, and oligomers in development for rare diseases will benefit from that. In addition, it is likely that far more extensive, sophisticated and longer term monitoring will be required of the new drugs after they are approved. That trend is already in evidence for new medicines. Nobody wants to see another Vioxx or

Avandia debacle, so more extensive post-marketing safety surveillance will become the rule rather than the exception.

The oligomer (or oligonucleotide, the terms are generally used interchangeably) community is optimistic about the future of these gene patches and desires transparency so that doctors, healthcare scientists, and consumers alike can become better informed and share the excitement.

Over the last few years, new societies have formed, like the Oligonucleotide Therapeutic Society, OTS, where scientists exchange latest information about the development of these patches. As these societies grow and the pace of progress speeds up, distilling the information overload down to manageable chunks for us all to consume will become a mighty task. Books, journals, television, and the Internet will all be harnessed in providing doctors, and you, with updates and advice.

In the future, not only will your doctors and their offices change to encompass the rapidly increasing amount of genetic data, but the drugs they prescribe as well as your hospital dispensaries and your local pharmacies, will change too. The regional warehouses and distribution networks that supply these pharmacies will also have to rapidly adapt to the new paradigm.

Pharmacies now stock a surprisingly small number of drugs – only about 30,000 discrete medicines, although many are made by multiple different manufacturers and in different strengths, bottle size, or formulations for different routes of administration. The medicines are often relatively inexpensive due to the tremendous technical advances in quality manufacturing. The original manufacturer of the first brand of a new drug can charge a premium price to recoup the enormous costs of development. The cost of manufacture of conventional medicines, especially pills, is modest in comparison to the new gene patches, which require many additional steps, some of which are quite complex, in their manufacture.

So today, pharmacy shelves are stocked with bottles and packets of pills which have been relatively inexpensive to manufacture. Pharmacies can afford to buy large quantities of them, each with long shelf lives. The pharmacy, retailer, distributor, and manufacturer can all benefit from bulk production, packing, purchasing, and shipping. Each pharmacy may have hundreds, even thousands, of patients on each drug, so they turn over their massive stock on a regular basis. Inventory control is vital to ensure they stock enough of the popular drugs to meet demand and not too much of the less popular medicines since shelf space is valuable.

The new oligomers will require development of a leaner and more efficient supply chain. The initial cost of manufacture will be significantly greater than today's blockbuster pills. As more manufacturers develop the capability and experience, and the raw materials – the chemical building blocks – become more plentiful, so the price of manufacture will fall. However, instead of each pharmacy having hundreds or thousands of patients on each of their drugs, each oligomer may only be appropriate for a very few highly select patients with the exact genetic mutation for which the oligomer has been designed. For some rare diseases, there may only be a handful of patients across the whole of the United States. Thus it would be totally impractical for every pharmacy to stock that oligomer.

Actually, these oligomers are unlikely initially to be dispensed by your neighborhood retail pharmacy at all. For some years after the first few oligomers have been approved, and others accelerate through development, these new gene patches are likely to be available only to select doctors. Perhaps they will work in special teams or hospitals with the skill to assess and monitor the disease being tackled and prevented.

The pharmacies of these hospitals are where the new oligomers will be delivered. The shipments will be quite small, so the supply and distribution will need to be more highly coordinated.

Some of the new oligomers may only be administered to handfuls of patients worldwide. So instead of the current system where manufacturing can occur in numerous countries around the globe, the new gene patches may only be made in one factory. Shipping overseas, meeting export and import requirements, and then getting from the port of entry in the destination country to any distant hospital will require considerably more sophisticated tracking and logistic support. There may be, for instance, more security than is currently the norm.

Gradually, a few hospitals will stock a small number of these new oligomers as vials of injectable product, or freeze dried powder for reconstitution at the time of administration. The first candidates for possible treatment with these gene patches will reflect the interest and expertise of the doctors at the institution. It may be the only hospital in that country, continent, or even the world dealing with that particular rare disease.

In time, many large hospital pharmacies will carry a large array of gene patch medicines. Each oligomer, though, will be for a small, select group of patients, with a variety of rare diseases or a unique genetic pattern for a more common disease. Perhaps the stock will be released to each hospital or clinic on a named patient basis, with responsibility for monitoring the products' longer term safety shared between the hospital-based doctor, the hospital pharmacy and the manufacturing company.

Initially, the new gene patches will be administered by the named hospital physician who cares for the disease in question. Only as experience is gained with these oligomers and their safety record becomes established over years will your primary care doctor be able to administer them. Even then the initial prescription may be made by a super specialist who will share the safety monitoring with your local doctor.

The vials of oligomers may start off at the regional center and then transfer on a named patient basis, to a local hospital or to your local doctor to administer them.

Imagine a world where oligomers are developed for just ten percent of the one in ten Americans with a rare disease, or one out of every one hundred patients. If your doctor has a list of three thousand patients, that means thirty patients (3000 divided by 100) will be receiving an oligomer once a month. If those who suffer from rare diseases return to the super specialist hospital every six months for shared care, your neighborhood doctor may need to store 180 vials of oligomers to cover the period between visits to the specialty center. That is certainly manageable in most offices and clinics.

Patient advocacy organizations may be able to help with the identification of patients. They may also have lists of the small number of hospitals where each new oligomer will be available. Thus they may play an even more important role in future, linking patient to hospital, and accelerating access to these new medicines.

In this possible future, the hospital where the super regional specialist works will be the site where the diagnosis, assessment, and initial treatment of a new patient with a suspected rare disease will take place. Once the disease has been stabilized, the patient will be referred to a neighborhood local hospital or doctor's office where the drug can be administered. Since many genetic diseases will be diagnosed at birth from the samples taken from a new baby, newborns will be referred to the regional hospital and this is where the new treatment will be explained to anxious parents. The baby will have no signs of the disease in question. Everyone's aim will be for that to remain the case.

Electronic medical records and bar coding of new drugs will become the norm. They will link the right patient to the right drug at the right dose, administered at the right time. It will automatically be confirmed as the drug is dispensed. As a baby grows and gains weight, the dose of a new oligomer will need to be adjusted and the cumulative dose of drug tracked. A new batch of stock will be ordered as existing stock is utilized, in good time for the next administration. Or a set of vials will be produced, sent to, and stored at the specialty hospital to be subsequently sent back to the local team. Much of that supply-tracking technology is in place now for existing drugs.

Summary

When you put all this information together, you get a clear picture of what medical practice will look like in the future, in terms of dispensing patches for your genes:

If your hospital specialist prescribes an oligomer, the hospital pharmacy will perform a verification check of your electronic medical record to confirm the oligomer you need, and the dose. The vials of freeze dried oligomers will be stored in the pharmacy or in the future may be transferred to your local doctor's office to be kept in a secure cabinet. Freeze dried product will have a much longer shelf life at varying temperatures and will therefore be far easier to store than already dissolved product, even in the same glass vials. As the vial is removed from the secure cabinet, it will trigger an automatic request to the manufacturer to start producing a new batch, like the system used in hotel minibars. Sterile saline will be injected into the vial and the oligomer will be reconstituted into solution. The vial will be bar coded, so it can be checked against your record to confirm that it is the right medicine for you. In fact, bar coding a vial of your personalized oligomer will allow it to be tracked from manufacturer, to distributor, to warehouse, to airport or trucking depot, to the hospital and onward to your doctor. All of these locations will have bar code reading equipment so that the vial of your oligomer can be tracked across time and space, much as a FedEx package is today.

Before your doctor administers your monthly dose, she will check that you have not reacted adversely to previous injections. Any adverse events you report may be transmitted back to the manufacturer, with that safety information being sent on to the FDA's safety reporting system. While each manufacturer will maintain a database about the safety of their oligomer, or oligomers, the FDA will keep anonymous detailed versions of all safety reports from all manufacturers and thus have a far more complete picture of the overall safety of the numerous types of gene patches already marketed or in development.

With the prescription of these new personalized gene patches comes a much greater chance of ensuring benefit and preventing harm. But the patches will be made on an almost individual basis and they will need to be shipped from manufacturer to the patient's hospital pharmacy directly by a far more sophisticated system than that employed today. From there, the oligomers may be transferred to a named doctor, close to the patient, who will share care with the instigating hospital specialist.

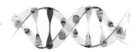

Chapter 11

To Infinity and Beyond

G ene patches are only part of how medicine will change in the next fifty years. If you think what I've described so far sounds like science-fiction, wait until I give you a peek at what else is possible.

After all, it's only been a bit more than forty years since we walked on the moon. Who would have thought that since then we would be able to hold a video conversation with friends or family on the other side of the world? Or that we could store the information from a set of encyclopedias on a hard drive the size of a pinhead? (That is still a lot bigger and a lot less information than is contained in the human genome!)

Over the next fifty years, medicine will change dramatically. Here are the top ten ways it will evolve:

10) More drugs will be delivered by inhalation.

I am a big proponent of aerosol delivery of drugs through the lungs and immediately into the bloodstream. In the past, inhaler devices have been relatively unsophisticated. But that is changing and soon, the first of many new systemic drugs should be approved for delivery by inhalation. Levadex, an anti-migraine drug developed by MAP Pharmaceuticals uses a more sophisticated inhaler device and has been used to deliver an old drug, dihydroergotamine, to those in the throes of a distressing migraine episode. But there are many more novel inhaler devices in development. The lungs have many built-in protections, specifically to prevent inhaled particles from getting into the body. We are getting cleverer at bypassing these defense mechanisms.

In another fifty years, more drugs that need to get into the bloodstream quickly (and avoid the liver which breaks most drugs down), will be delivered by one of the next generation of inhalers. They will completely surpass the old press-and-breath metered dose inhalers first introduced in the 1950s, that many patients with lung diseases still use today. The new devices will also deliver better medicines, faster and more effectively to those with lung disease. Until smoking is outlawed, that will always be a large number.

9) Implanted devices will include a slow-release drug that reduces the body's attempts to attack the implant.

Many stents used today for opening up blocked arteries already carry these slow-release drugs. But the number and variety of implanted devices, often inserted in an acute situation to rapidly reverse a crisis and before long-term damage can be done, will greatly increase. This will require more regulatory flexibility than seen today as the effects of the therapy, both good and bad, may be shared by drug and device. Indeed, great changes within the regulatory framework for new medicines and devices will be necessary to ensure the Golden Age of Medicine is not hampered by outdated and obstructive bureaucracy.

8) Regenerative medicine will reduce the need to obtain replacements for failing organs from sudden death victims. Replacements will instead be grown in the laboratory.

Stem cells and regenerative medicine are on the verge of coming of age. It will be possible to repair damaged organs, even replace missing ones, by the insertion of stem cells with the potential to develop into specialized cells of the organ or body part. Already it is possible to grow some body parts outside of the body and then introduce them. New bladders are being created experimentally by the Wake Forest Institute for Regenerative Medicine in North Carolina. There, over two dozen children and young adults born with defective bladders have already had new laboratory-grown ones implanted. They have even built kidneys in the laboratory, that when implanted into animals, have produced urine. But the field will evolve rapidly with specialist companies developing the right growth factor supplements to help the stem cells develop into a new organ, a kidney, a liver or skin. So if you have a serious injury in a car crash, your damaged parts will be replaced using the power of regenerative medicine.

This will be important, because as our life expectancy increases (it's already up by eleven years for men and twelve for women just in the last four decades), many more people will work into their seventies and eighties. As their organs, joints or tissues age, they may need replacements, and it will be much easier to get them in fifty years. This will help the aging population remain more mentally and physically active.

7) Fully portable electronic medical records will be commonplace.

The records will be initiated when you are born and will have information loaded on at every healthcare encounter with your doctor, your local hospital, the specialist hospital, your pharmacy, your dentist and your optician. Each will be able to enter new data and view existing data relevant to their practice. This will help you to receive faster and safer care. Maybe the information will be stored on a microchip worn as a locket or on a wrist strap. We may even have the option to keep these chips implanted under the skin as we do already with our pets. That is the surest way to keep you and your record united.

6) Small hospitals with community ties will replace the current huge university-based teaching centers.

Huge mega hospitals that treat thousands of patients in big, often university-based, teaching centers will become a thing of the past. Imagine a world where Seattle Grace, of *Grey's Anatomy,* is replaced by the much smaller medical facilities of *Private Practice.* There will be smaller units built with much closer links to community-based health-care teams. There will be smaller mobile, or fixed, operating "rooms." These units will be able to operate at a much higher efficiency than today's operating room and will be open 18, or even 24 hours a day, at a fraction of today's costs, with support staff preparing patients.

5) Surgery will be performed remotely on a routine basis – and most surgery will be microsurgery and use a microscope.

Surgery will routinely be performed by surgeons who are remote from the operating table using sophisticated, microscopic video cameras and minute tools worked robotically over the internet. This is already possible and has been done, though it hasn't been widely publicized. Let's say the best hand surgeon in the world is in France and you are in Chicago. You will be able to get her to work on you in Chicago without leaving her home in Paris. This will have many benefits, including democratizing health care so that everyone has access to top surgeons.

In-person surgery will still be performed, but there will be a stronger focus on microsurgery. And the operations will be much less invasive, so the post-operative recovery will be much faster with many more patients able to return home on the same day, and back to work within a few days.

4) A spit swab for genome sequencing will replace the heel prick that is done when a baby is born today.

Since a blood test at birth is far less revealing than genetic testing, insurance companies will cover the cost of this test. The outlay will be a fraction of today's prices, due to increasing automation and competition. The insurance companies will have embraced the need to provide coverage for diseases that are identified and will help you, through your doctor, avoid many of the triggers and adverse behaviors that contribute to illness today.

With more in-depth information about the genetic risks of various ailments, health, and how to sustain it, will be taught better in school. The result will be that our children and grandchildren will make better lifestyle choices for themselves than today's overweight, unhealthy population.

3) Blood tests will disappear.

A whole new series of disease monitoring devices and measurements will be available. Many diseases currently untreatable, or other diseases where the monitoring of the disease's effects are crude, will have new biomarkers identified. These new methods will be more sensitive, more predictive and more specific than those available today. In addition they will be less invasive. Today's blood tests will be replaced by collecting a urine sample, breathing into an analyzer, or taking a hair sample. The machines needed to monitor these biomarkers will be small, portable and easy to operate, so that management of many more diseases will be overseen by your primary care practitioner, or internist, in your own neighborhood. The need for regular checkups, even for the few diseases where effective therapy may still be lacking, will involve less travel, upheaval, stress and cost for you and your family.

2) New bugs will be stopped dead in their tracks.

Infectious diseases will be tackled on a much faster basis.

In the last century we have made remarkable progress already against communicable disease. But there are still some microbial enemies pitted against us that have yet to be beaten back. Oligomers will play an important but marginal role in this battle. The oligomers will be too expensive for everyday use, but they will be ideal for rare, lethal diseases or the emergence of multi-drug resistant strains.

Big hospitals heretofore have been a major breeding ground for new bugs. The small number that will remain to undertake heroic surgery or care for desperately ill patients with all the sophisticated life support systems will be linked to special laboratories. When a new infection is discovered, almost on an individual patient level, samples of the infection will be examined, the bug identified and the sequence of its RNA determined. Oligomers against that bug will be rapidly developed and the bug will literally be stopped dead in its tracks. Lethal hospital acquired infections and outbreaks of fatal pandemics will be contained and defeated within a few days with the use of fast response teams aided by scrupulous quarantine and impeccable logistical support.

1) Gene patch therapy will be superseded by gene replacement therapy.

The healing powers of oligomers will only be a start. The miraculous results they get will only whet researchers' appetites so that a

Band-Aid will no longer be enough. Scientists will want to be able to provide a full cure. And the only full cure that will truly work for an untreatable rare disease will be replacing the faulty gene that created it. As societies, we will struggle with the ethics of inserting new genes and removing less favorable ones. There will be a tremendous fear of designer babies. And certain countries where boy babies are preferred may go through some upheaval, as too many baby boys will lead to a lot of lonely old men.

But the potential to fully heal the millions of people with rare diseases will be so powerful that it will overcome the issues that stem from this new technology.

As to what will be the more traditional procedure, the gene patch, it will live up to its full potential. Tomorrow's gene patches will be highly targeted drugs that will bind to up to thirty letters or so of our messenger RNA as it peels off the three billion letters of our genome.

The variety of chemistries being used and the number of companies developing these gene patches will have dramatically increased. The growth of this industry will accelerate as the first few gene patches are approved and the regulators become more familiar with the technology and its strengths and weaknesses. Blockbuster drugs will slowly decline in number and a large number of far more personalized drugs will be manufactured. This will be true of drugs in general, not just the wave of RNA targeting oligomers. They will all be much more targeted to you and your disease.

Your own doctor will be far more involved in delivering the oligomers to you than with previous medicines, and monitoring your continued wellness throughout your life. The oligomers will be tracked even down to the individual vial with replacement supplies being generated by the manufacturers on an individual patient basis.

Careful follow up of these gene patches, and larger, longer, more detailed safety follow up of all drugs, not just oligomers, will be rigorously enforced.

******

One final note: To make things easier to understand, I have simplified the truth about rare diseases and how they can be treated by gene patch medicine. Unfortunately, the story is a lot more complex than I have suggested. I'd like to take the last few paragraphs of this book to give you a fuller picture of how things work.

Not everyone with even the same rare disease has the same genetic makeup. Duchenne muscular dystrophy for instance. It has many different genetic variations that lead to the lack of the vital dystrophin in the muscles. Only about 85% of DMD patients have a genetic mutation that can be treated by skipping an exon, and even for those, there are twenty or more different exon targets, one or more of which may need to be skipped to restore the RNA reading frame.

If your son is diagnosed with DMD, you will need to know exactly which one of the hundreds of different genetic mutations he has, and therefore which of the numerous gene patches he should be given. Some patients may need more than one patch! Research is already under way on that topic.

The companies developing the DMD oligomers believe their oligomers generate new, functioning dystrophin for the most common form of DMD. Both companies, Prosensa and Sarepta have other oligomers currently in development personalized to skip other exons for different genetic variants of DMD. The exact genetic profile of the individual must be very carefully characterized to ensure that the new gene patches work and apply themselves, like a Band-Aid, to exactly the right bit of the molecular message, the mRNA.

More recently both companies have reported clinical benefit from their initial exon 51 skipping programs, demonstrated by an improvement in walking, albeit over just six minutes.

But will the new dystrophin now being detected in the early clinical studies replace the missing protein in all muscles, and at the same rate?

DMD affects all muscles, limbs, breathing muscles of the chest, back muscles supporting the spine, and even the heart muscle. It also has adverse consequences on the development and functioning of the brain. We still do not know if the missing dystrophin in the chest or heart muscles can be replaced, and the breathing and heart functions preserved. And we don't know for sure whether the brain will also benefit too from the functional, but shortened dystrophin generated by these new oligomers.

And then there's the question of timing. Will the gene patch work on all these organs if it is given to the growing fetus during pregnancy for the full benefits to accrue?

There is still much work to be done as we learn about these new gene patch medicines. As we answer one question, three more pop up. Today's exciting scientific breakthroughs will seem mundane as we delve more deeply into the genome to try to better design and target the next generation of gene patches.

Personalized medicine is here to stay, in your doctor's office, at your local hospital, at the regional, national and university centers as well as on some bigger pharmacy shelves. With this new focus, comes an ability to better diagnose, monitor and treat disease effectively and safely. We will also be able to predict and prevent future ill health and promote well-being.

How quickly society grasps these new paradigms remains to be seen, but many are ready and willing now, not least those patients and their families with rare diseases for whom RNA targeting oligomers brings hope of effective management, if not a "cure" for their disease. In comparison to the advances over the last five thousand years, the advances likely in the next fifty have the potential to transform our society like nothing before. We are entering a Golden Age of Medicine. One day soon you will be able to *Defy Your DNA*.

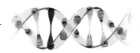

Appendix A

Top 20 Drugs in 2010 in the U.S. by Annual Sales
(Data From Companies)

	Drug	Manufacturer (U.S., EU, Japan)	Annual spend	Indication
1	Lipitor	Pfizer U.S.	$12.7 Billion	High cholesterol
2	Plavix	Bristol-Myers Squibb (BMS) U.S. & Sanofi Aventis EU	$8.8 Billion	Heart disease
3	Remicade	Johnson & Johnson U.S., Merck U.S., Mitsubishi J & Tanabe J	$8.0 Billion	Rheumatoid arthritis
4	Advair	GlaxoSmithKline EU	$8.0 Billion	Asthma, COPD
5	Enbrel	Amgen U.S., Pfizer U.S., Takeda J	$7.4 Billion	Rheumatoid arthritis
6	Avastin	Roche EU	$6.8 Billion	Cancer
7	Abilify	Otsuka J, BMS U.S.	$6.8 Billion	Schizophrenia,
8	Rituxan	Roche EU	$6.7 Billion	Lymphoma, Leukemia
9	Humira	Abbott U.S.	$6.5 Billion	Rheumatoid Arthritis
10	Diovan	Novartis EU	$6.1 Billion	Hypertension
11	Crestor	Astra Zeneca EU, Shionoggi J	$6.0 Billion	Cholesterol
12	Lovenox	Sanofi Aventis EU	$5.8 Billion	Anticoagulant
13	Seroquel	Astra Zeneca EU	$5.6 Billion	Schizophrenia
14	Herceptin	Roche EU	$5.5 Billion	Breast Cancer
15	Nexium	Astra Zeneca EU	$5.0 Billion	Heartburn
16	Zyprexa	Eli Lilly U.S.	$4.9 Billion	Schizophrenia
17	Singulair	Merck U.S.	$4.9 Billion	Asthma, allergy
18	Lantus	Sanofi Aventis EU	$4.7 Billion	Diabetes
19	Actos	Takeda J	$4.5 Billion	Diabetes
20	Copaxone	Teva Israel, Sanofi Aventis EU	$4.0 Billion	Multiple sclerosis

Appendix B

FDA Orphan Drug Approvals
in First Nine Months of 2010

Product/ Company	Indication	Month approved	Division	NDA/ BLA
Dalfampridine/ Acorda	Multiple sclerosis	Jan	DNP	NDA
Collagenase/ Auxilium	Dupuytren's contracture	Feb	DPARP	BLA
Velaglucerase/ Shire	Gaucher's disease	Feb	DGP	NDA
Carglumic acid/ Orphan Europe	NAGS (N -acetylglu-tamate synthetase) deficiency	March	DGP	NDA
Alglucosidase alfa/ Genzyme	Late-onset Pompe disease	May	DGP	BLA
Glycopyrrulate/ Shionogi	Drooling in children with neurological disease	July	DNP	NDA
Pegloticase/ Savient	Chronic (unrespon-sive) gout	September	DPARP	BLA

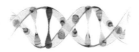

Glossary of Terms

Many of these terms are taken from the public "Talking Glossary of Genetic Terms" available from the National Human Genome Research Institute at http://genome.gov/glossary.cfm

ACGT: The acronym for the four types of bases found in a DNA molecule: adenine (A), cytosine (C), guanine (G), and thymine (T). A DNA molecule consists of two strands wound around each other, with each strand held together by bonds between the bases. Adenine pairs with thymine, and cytosine pairs with guanine. The sequence of bases in a portion of a DNA molecule, called a gene, carries the instructions needed to assemble a protein.

Allele: One of two or more versions of a gene. An individual inherits two alleles for each gene, one from each parent. If the two alleles are the same, the individual is homozygous for that gene. If the alleles are different, the individual is heterozygous. Though the term "allele" was originally used to describe variation among genes, it now also refers to variation among non-coding DNA sequences.

Amino Acid: 20 different molecules used to build proteins. Proteins consist of one or more chains of amino acids called polypeptides. The sequence of the amino acid chain causes the polypeptide

213

to fold into a shape that is biologically active. The amino acid sequences of proteins are encoded in the genes.

Antisense: The non-coding DNA strand of a gene. A cell uses antisense DNA strand as a template for producing messenger RNA (mRNA) that directs the synthesis of a protein. Antisense can also refer to a method for silencing genes. To silence a target gene, a second gene is introduced that produces an mRNA complementary to that produced from the target gene. These two mRNAs can interact to form a double-stranded structure that cannot be used to direct protein synthesis.

Autosomal dominance: A pattern of inheritance characteristic of some genetic diseases. "Autosomal" means that the gene in question is located on one of the numbered, or non-sex, chromosomes. "Dominant" means that a single copy of the disease-associated mutation is enough to cause the disease. This is in contrast to a recessive disorder, where two copies of the mutation are needed to cause the disease. Huntington's disease is a common example of an autosomal dominant genetic disorder.

Bacteria: Small single-celled organisms. Bacteria are found almost everywhere on Earth and are vital to the planet's ecosystems. Some species can live under extreme conditions of temperature and pressure. The human body is full of bacteria, and in fact is estimated to contain more bacterial cells than human cells. Most bacteria in the body are harmless, and some are even helpful. A relatively small number of species cause disease.

Base pair: The two chemical bases bonded to one another forming a "rung of the DNA ladder." The DNA molecule consists of two strands that wind around each other like a twisted ladder. Each strand has a backbone made of alternating sugar (deoxyribose) and phosphate groups. Attached to each sugar is one of four bases--adenine (A), cytosine (C), guanine (G), or thymine (T). The two strands are held together by hydrogen bonds between the bases, with adenine forming a base pair with thymine, and cytosine forming a base pair with guanine.

BRCA1 and BRCA2: The first two genes found to be associated with an inherited form of cancer. Both genes normally act as tumor suppressors, meaning that they help regulate cell division. When these genes are rendered inactive due to mutation, uncontrolled cell growth results, leading to breast cancer. Women with mutations in either gene have a much higher risk for developing breast cancer than women without mutations in the genes.

Carcinogen: An agent with the capacity to cause cancer in humans. Carcinogens may be natural, such as aflatoxin, which is produced by a fungus and sometimes found on stored grains, or manmade, such as asbestos or tobacco smoke. Carcinogens work by interacting with a cell's DNA and inducing genetic mutations.

Carrier: An individual who carries and is capable of passing on a genetic mutation associated with a disease and may or may not display disease symptoms. Carriers are associated with diseases inherited as recessive traits. In order to have the disease, an individual must have inherited mutated alleles from both parents. An individual having one normal allele and one mutated allele does not have the disease. Two carriers may produce children with the disease.

Cell: The basic building block of living things. All cells can be sorted into one of two groups: eukaryotes and prokaryotes. A eukaryote has a nucleus and membrane-bound organelles, while a prokaryote does not. Plants and animals are made of numerous eukaryotic cells, while many microbes, such as bacteria, consist of single prokaryote cells. An adult human body is estimated to contain between 10 and 100 trillion cells.

Cell membrane (also called plasma membrane)**:** Found in all cells and separates the interior of the cell from the outside environment. The cell membrane consists of a lipid bilayer that is semipermeable. The cell membrane regulates the transport of materials entering and exiting the cell.

Chromosome: An organized package of DNA found in the nucleus of the cell. Different organisms have different numbers of chromosomes. Humans have 23 pairs of chromosomes--22 pairs of numbered chromosomes, called autosomes, and one pair of sex chromosomes, XX (female) or XY (male). Each parent contributes one chromosome to each pair so that offspring get half of their chromosomes from their mother and half from their father.

Codon: A trinucleotide sequence of DNA or RNA that corresponds to a specific amino acid. The genetic code describes the relationship between the sequence of DNA bases (A, C, G, and T) in a gene and the corresponding protein sequence that it encodes. The cell reads the sequence of the gene in groups of three bases. There are 64 different codons: 61 specify amino acids while the remaining three are used as stop signals

Congenital conditions: Those present from birth. Birth defects are described as being congenital. They can be caused by a genetic mutation, an unfavorable environment in the uterus, or a combination of both factors.

Copy number variation (CNV): When the number of copies of a particular gene varies from one individual to the next. Following the completion of the Human Genome Project, it became apparent that the genome experiences gains and losses of genetic material. The extent to which copy number variation contributes to human disease is not yet known. It has long been recognized that some cancers are associated with elevated copy numbers of particular genes.

Cystic fibrosis: A hereditary disease characterized by faulty digestion, breathing problems, respiratory infections from mucus buildup, and the loss of salt in sweat. The disease is caused by mutations in a single gene and is inherited as an autosomal recessive trait, meaning that an affected individual must inherit two mutated copies of the gene to get the disease. In the past, cystic fibrosis was almost always fatal in childhood. Today, however, patients commonly live to be 30 years or older.

Cytoplasm: The gelatinous liquid that fills the inside of a cell. It is composed of water, salts, and various organic molecules. Some intracellular organelles, such the nucleus and mitochondria, are enclosed by membranes that separate them from the cytoplasm.

Diabetes mellitus: A disease characterized by an inability to make or use the hormone insulin. Insulin is needed by cells to metabolize glucose, the body's main source of chemical energy. Type I diabetes, also called insulin-dependent diabetes mellitus, is usually caused by an autoimmune destruction of insulin-producing cells. Type II diabetes, also called non-insulin-dependent diabetes mellitus, occurs when cells become resistant to the effects of insulin.

Diploid: a cell or organism that has paired chromosomes, one from each parent. In humans, cells other than human sex cells, are diploid and have 23 pairs of chromosomes. Human sex cells (egg and sperm cells) contain a single set of chromosomes and are known as haploid.

DNA (Deoxyribonucleic Acid): the chemical name for the molecule that carries genetic instructions in all living things. The DNA molecule consists of two strands that wind around one another to form a shape known as a double helix. Each strand has a backbone made of alternating sugar (deoxyribose) and phosphate groups. Attached to each sugar is one of four bases--adenine (A), cytosine (C), guanine

(G), and thymine (T). The two strands are held together by bonds between the bases; adenine bonds with thymine, and cytosine bonds with guanine. The sequence of the bases along the backbones serves as instructions for assembling protein and RNA molecules.

DNA sequencing: A laboratory technique used to determine the exact sequence of bases (A, C, G, and T) in a DNA molecule. The DNA base sequence carries the information a cell needs to assemble protein and RNA molecules. DNA sequence information is important to scientists investigating the functions of genes. The technology of DNA sequencing was made faster and less expensive as a part of the Human Genome Project.

Duplication: A type of mutation that involves the production of one or more copies of a gene or region of a chromosome. Gene and chromosome duplications occur in all organisms, though they are especially prominent among plants. Gene duplication is an important mechanism by which evolution occurs.

Enzyme: A biological catalyst and is almost always a protein. It speeds up the rate of a specific chemical reaction in the cell. The enzyme is not destroyed during the reaction and is used over and over again. A cell contains thousands of different types of enzyme molecules, each specific to a particular chemical reaction.

Exon: The portion of a gene that codes for amino acids. In the cells of plants and animals, most gene sequences are broken up by one or more DNA sequences called introns. The parts of the gene sequence that are expressed in the protein are called exons, because they are expressed, while the parts of the gene sequence that are not expressed in the protein are called introns, because they come in between--or interfere with--the exons.

Founder effect: The reduction in genetic variation that results when a small subset of a large population is used to establish a new colony. The new population may be very different from the original population, both in terms of its genotypes and phenotypes. In some cases, the founder effect plays a role in the emergence of new species.

Frameshift mutation: A type of mutation involving the insertion or deletion of a nucleotide in which the number of deleted base pairs is not divisible by three. "Divisible by three" is important because the cell reads a gene in groups of three bases. Each group of three bases corresponds to one of 20 different amino acids used to build a protein. If a mutation disrupts this reading frame, then the entire DNA sequence following the mutation will be read incorrectly.

Gene: The basic physical unit of inheritance. Genes are passed from parents to offspring and contain the information needed to specify traits. Genes are arranged, one after another, on structures called chromosomes. A chromosome contains a single, long DNA molecule, only a portion of which corresponds to a single gene. Humans have approximately 25,000 genes arranged on their chromosomes.

Gene expression: The process by which the information encoded in a gene is used to direct the assembly of a protein molecule. The cell reads the sequence of the gene in groups of three bases. Each group of three bases (codon) corresponds to one of 20 different amino acids used to build the protein.

Gene mapping: The process of establishing the locations of genes on the chromosomes. Early gene maps used linkage analysis. The closer two genes are to each other on the chromosome, the more likely it is that they will be inherited together. By following inheritance patterns, the relative positions of genes can be determined. More recently, scientists have used recombinant DNA (rDNA) techniques to establish the actual physical locations of genes on the chromosomes.

Genome: The entire set of genetic instructions found in a cell. In humans, the genome consists of 23 pairs of chromosomes, found in the nucleus, as well as a small chromosome found in the cells' mitochondria. These chromosomes, taken together, contain approximately 3 billion bases of DNA sequence.

Genome-wide association study (GWAS): An approach used in genetics research to associate specific genetic variations with particular diseases. The method involves scanning the genomes from many different people and looking for genetic markers that can be used to predict the presence of a disease. Once such genetic markers are identified, they can be used to understand how genes contribute to the disease and develop better prevention and treatment strategies.

Genomics: Refers to the study of the entire genome of an organism whereas genetics refers to the study of a particular gene.

Genotype: An individual's collection of genes. The term also can refer to the two alleles inherited for a particular gene. The genotype is expressed when the information encoded in the genes' DNA is used to make protein and RNA molecules. The expression of the genotype contributes to the individual's observable traits, called the phenotype.

Heterozygous: Where an individual inherits different forms of a particular gene from each parent. A heterozygous genotype contrasts to a homozygous genotype, where an individual inherits identical forms of a particular gene from each parent.

Homozygous: Where an individual inherits the same alleles for a particular gene from both parents.

The Human Genome Project: An international project that mapped and sequenced the entire human genome. Completed in April 2003, data from the project are freely available to researchers and others interested in genetics and human health.

Intron: A portion of a gene that does not code for amino acids. In the cells of plants and animals, most gene sequences are broken up by one or more introns. The parts of the gene sequence that are expressed in the protein are called exons, because they are expressed, while the parts of the gene sequence that are not expressed in the protein are called introns, because they come in between the exons

Messenger RNA (mRNA): A single-stranded RNA molecule that is complementary to one of the DNA strands of a gene. The mRNA is an RNA version of the gene that leaves the cell nucleus and moves to the cytoplasm where proteins are made. During protein synthesis, an organelle called a ribosome moves along the mRNA, reads its base sequence, and uses the genetic code to translate each three-base triplet, or codon, into its corresponding amino acid.

Mitochondria: Membrane-bound cell organelles (mitochondrion, singular) that generate most of the chemical energy needed to power the cell's biochemical reactions. Mitochondria contain their own small chromosomes. Generally, mitochondria, and therefore mitochondrial DNA, are inherited only from the mother

Monomer: The simplest unit, of a repeating sequence of similar units, of a polymer.

Mutation: A change in a DNA sequence. Mutations can result from DNA copying mistakes made during cell division, exposure to ionizing radiation, exposure to chemicals called mutagens, or infection by viruses. Germ line mutations occur in the eggs and sperm and can be passed on to offspring, while somatic mutations occur in body cells and are not passed on.

Nonsense mutation: The substitution of a single base pair that leads to the appearance of a stop codon where previously there was a codon specifying an amino acid. The presence of this premature stop codon results in the production of a shortened, and likely nonfunctional, protein.

Nucleotide: The basic building block of nucleic acids. RNA and DNA are polymers made of long chains of nucleotides. A nucleotide consists of a sugar molecule (either ribose in RNA or deoxyribose in DNA) attached to a phosphate group and a nitrogen-containing base. The bases used in DNA are adenine (A), cytosine (C), guanine (G), and thymine (T). In RNA, the base uracil (U) takes the place of thymine.

Oligomer: A molecule that consists of a relatively small and specifiable number of monomers.

Oligonucleotide: Any molecule that contains a small number of nucleotide units connected by phosphodiester linkages between (usually) the 3′ position of one nucleotide and the 5′ position of the adjacent one. The number of nucleotide units in these small single-stranded nucleic acids (usually DNA) is variable but often in the range of 6 to 24 (hexamer to 24mer).

Oncogene: A mutated gene that contributes to the development of a cancer. In their normal, unmutated state, oncogenes are called proto-oncogenes, and they play roles in the regulation of cell division. Some oncogenes work like putting your foot down on the accelerator of a car, pushing a cell to divide. Other oncogenes work like removing your foot from the brake while parked on a hill, also causing the cell to divide.

Open reading frame: A portion of a DNA molecule that, when translated into amino acids, contains no stop codons. The genetic code reads DNA sequences in groups of three base pairs each being a codon).

Peptide: One or more amino acids linked by chemical bonds. The term also refers to the type of chemical bond that joins the amino acids together. A series of linked amino acids is a polypeptide. The cell's proteins are made from one or more polypeptides.

Personalized medicine: An emerging practice of medicine that uses an individual's genetic profile to guide decisions made in regard to the prevention, diagnosis, and treatment of disease. Knowledge of a patient's genetic profile can help doctors select the proper medication or therapy and administer it using the proper dose or regimen. Personalized medicine is being advanced through data from the Human Genome Project.

Pharmacogenomics: A branch of pharmacology concerned with using DNA and amino acid sequence data to inform drug development and testing. An important application of pharmacogenomics is correlating individual genetic variation with drug responses.

Phenotype: An individual's observable traits, such as height, eye color, and blood type. The genetic contribution to the phenotype is called the genotype. Some traits are largely determined by the genotype, while other traits are largely determined by environmental factors.

Plasma membrane: See cell membrane

Point mutation: When a single base pair is altered. Point mutations can have one of three effects. First, the base substitution can be a silent mutation where the altered codon corresponds to the same amino acid. Second, the base substitution can be a missense mutation where the altered codon corresponds to a different amino acid. Or third, the base substitution can be a nonsense mutation where the altered codon corresponds to a stop signal.

Proteins: An important class of molecules found in all living cells. A protein is composed of one or more long chains of amino acids, the sequence of which corresponds to the DNA sequence of the gene that encodes it. Proteins play a variety of roles in the cell, including structural (cytoskeleton), mechanical (muscle), biochemical (enzymes), and cell signaling (hormones). Proteins are also an essential part of diet.

Recessive: A quality found in the relationship between two versions of a gene. Individuals receive one version of a gene, called an allele, from each parent. If the alleles are different, the dominant allele will be expressed, while the effect of the other allele, called recessive, is masked. In the case of a recessive genetic disorder, an individual must inherit two copies of the mutated allele in order for the disease to be present.

Ribosome: A cellular particle made of RNA and protein that serves as the site for protein synthesis in the cell. The ribosome reads the sequence of the messenger RNA (mRNA) and, using the genetic code, translates the sequence of RNA bases into a sequence of amino acids.

Ribonucleic acid (RNA): A molecule similar to DNA. Unlike DNA, RNA is single-stranded. An RNA strand has a backbone made of alternating sugar (ribose) and phosphate groups. Attached to each sugar is one of four bases--adenine (A), uracil (U), cytosine (C), or guanine (G). Different types of RNA exist in the cell: messenger RNA (mRNA), ribosomal RNA (rRNA), and transfer RNA (tRNA). More recently microRNA has been found to be involved in regulating gene expression.

Sex linked: A trait in which a gene is located on a sex chromosome. In humans, the term generally refers to traits that are influenced by genes on the X chromosome. This is because the X chromosome is large and contains many more genes than the smaller Y chromosome. In a sex-linked disease, such as Duchenne muscular dystrophy, it is usually males who are affected because they have a single copy of X chromosome that carries the mutation. In females the effect of the mutation may be masked by the second healthy copy of the X chromosome.

Single nucleotide polymorphisms (SNPs): A type of polymorphism involving variation of a single base pair. Scientists are studying how single nucleotide polymorphisms, or SNPs (pronounced "snips"), in the human genome correlate with disease, drug response, and other phenotypes.

Transcription: The process of making an RNA copy of a gene sequence. This copy, called a messenger RNA (mRNA) molecule, leaves the cell nucleus and enters the cytoplasm, where it directs the synthesis of the protein, which it encodes.

Translation: The process of translating the sequence of a messenger RNA (mRNA) molecule to a sequence of amino acids during protein synthesis. The genetic code describes the relationship between the sequence of base pairs in a gene and the corresponding amino acid sequence that it encodes. In the cell cytoplasm, the ribosome reads the sequence of the mRNA in groups of three bases to assemble the protein.

X-linked: See sex linked

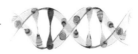

Bibliography

Books

Chiu LS. When a Gene Makes you Smell Like a Fish... and Other Tales about the Genes in Your Body (Oxford University Press)

Colby B. Outsmart Your Genes (Perigee)

Collins FS. The Language of Life (Harper Collins)

Davies K. The $1,000 Genome (Free Press)

Engel C. Wild Health: How Animals Keep Themselves Well and What We Can Learn From Them. (Weidenfeld and Nicolson)

Field MJ and Boat TF (Eds) – The Institute of Medicine. Rare Diseases and Orphan Products (National Academies Press)

Fields S and Johnston M. Genetic Twists of Fate (MIT Press)

Hanson W. The Edge of Medicine (Palgrave MacMillan)

Preston R. The Hot Zone (Anchor Books)

Schimpff SC. The Future of Medicine (Thomas Nelson)

Scientific journals

Journal of RNAi and Gene Silencing [http://libpubmedia.co.uk/RNAiJ/RNAiJHome.htm]

Nature Biotechnology [http://www.nature.com/nbt/index.html]

Neuromuscular Disorders [http://www.nmd-journal.com]

Nucleic Acid Therapeutics [http://www.liebertpub.com/NAT]

Pharmacogenomics and Personalized
Medicine [http://www.dovepress.com/
pharmacogenomics-and-personalized-medicine-journal]

Scientific papers

Cirak S, Arechavala-Gomeza V, Guglieri M et al. Exon skipping and
dystrophin restoration in Duchenne Muscular Dystrophy
patients after systemic phosphorodiamidate morpholino
oligomer treatment. Lancet 2011; 378: 595-605

FDA. Driving Biomedical Innovation: initiatives to Improve Products
for Patients. October 2011 @ www.fda.gov/innovation

Kole R, Krainer A, Altman S. RNA therapeutics: beyond RNA
interference and antisense oligonucleotides. (Nature Reviews
Drug Discovery 2012)

Schubert D, Levin AA, Kornbrust D et al. The Oligonucleotide
Safety Working Group [Editorial]. Nucleic Acid Technology
2012; 22(4): 211-212

Wood MJA, Gait MJ, Yin H. RNA-targeted splice-correction
therapy for neuromuscular disease. (Brain 2010)

Organizations

NORD: http://www.rarediseases.org

EURORDIS: http://www.eurordis.org

Muscular Dystrophy Association: http://mda.org

Parent Project Muscular Dystrophy: http: //www.parentprojectmd.org

Personalized Medicine Coalition: http://www.personalizedmedicine coalition.org

Cure Duchenne: http://www.cureduchenne.org

Action Duchenne (UK): http://www.actionduchenne.org

Progeria Research Foundation: http://www.progeriaresearch.org

23andMe: https://www.23andme.com

deCODE: http://www.decode.com

General Genetics Corporation: http://www.ggcdna.com

Alnylam: http://www.alnylam.com

Isis Pharmaceuticals: http: //www.isispharm.com

MAP Pharmaceuticals: http://www.mappharma.com

Prosensa: http://www.prosensa.eu

Sarepta Therapeutics: http://www.sareptatherapeutics.com

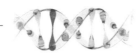

Index

www.defyyourdnabook.com

www.facebook.com/defyyourdnabook